SOFT TISSUE MASSAGE FOR PAIN RELIEF

SOFT TISSUE MASSAGE
FOR PAIN RELIEF

*How You Can
Massage Away
the Pain from
37 Health
Conditions*

BERNARD SCHATZ, P.T.

HAMPTON ROADS
PUBLISHING COMPANY, INC.

Cover design by Steve Amarillo
Cover art by Eyewire
Interior drawings by Bernard Schatz
Author photo by Becky Lutz

For information write:

Hampton Roads Publishing Company, Inc.
1125 Stoney Ridge Road
Charlottesville, VA 22902

434-296-2772
fax: 434-296-5096
e-mail: hrpc@hrpub.com
www.hrpub.com

If you are unable to order this book from your local
bookseller, you may order directly from the publisher.
Call 1-800-766-8009, toll-free.

Library of Congress Catalog Card Number: 2001094079
ISBN 1-57174-264-6
10 9 8 7 6 5 4 3 2 1
Printed on acid-free paper in Canada

This book was written for body and headache pain sufferers who have been examined by doctors, received their treatments . . . *and continue to suffer*.

It is dedicated to the many who somehow get through each day of pain. You are true heroes.

Table of Contents

Foreword

The words "pain relief" actually can mean either of two things: *temporary* relief from pain (because the treatment dealt only with symptoms) or *permanent* relief (because the treatment dealt not with symptoms but with causes). This book is about treating the cause and thus obtaining permanent relief.

Treating the body is an adventure. There is so much that is unknown. The human body is so complex. Every individual is so different, so unique, that it is a constant learning process to treat the body.

For a practitioner, the stress is terrible when someone comes to you in severe pain. We are surrounded by a great human tragedy. Millions of people suffer severe, unremitting body and headache pain. Their suffering is needless, avoidable, and inexcusable. But the sense of excitement, of adventure, is still there, especially with the expectation that the key to that person's return to health lies somewhere within that bundle of tissues before you.

And there is no greater thrill of discovery than when that key is found!

Take a moment to take the following true-or-false quiz before reading this book. After reading the book, please review the quiz and consider how your answers may change now. . . .

1. You can assume the doctor dealing with your body or headache pain is intelligent, creative, and open to fresh ideas.　　　　T　or　F

2. You can be confident your doctor examined you in a way that determined the cause of your body or headache pain, and allowed enough time to examine you carefully and thoroughly.　　　　T　or　F

3. You can trust everything your doctor tells you about your body or headache pain.　　　　T　or　F

4. You should treat your doctor with great respect, awe, admiration, and deference regarding his or her care of your ongoing body or headache pain.　　T　or　F

5. Body and headache pain are best treated with drugs, surgery, or a visit to a psychiatrist.　　　　T　or　F

6. Names such as fibromyalgia, migraine and carpal tunnel syndrome explain the cause of your pain.　　T　or　F

7. Migraine, carpal tunnel syndrome, and fibromyalgia have nothing in common.　　　　T　or　F

8. Tendons swell easily.　　　　T　or　F

9. Pain management centers will treat your body or headache pain.　　　　T　or　F

10. You should always believe your doctor when he tells you that nothing more can be done for your body or headache pain.　　　　T　or　F

If you answered true to any of these questions, you need to read the book carefully. But before you do, here are some typical questions I get from new pain patients, and my answers.

Q: You often use the phrase "body and headache pain." Why aren't you more specific and say migraine, osteoarthritis, or fibromyalgia?

A: Millions of people suffer severe, unremitting, and crippling pain. Doctors are able to determine the cause of only a small fraction of this vast ocean of pain. For example, doctors can diagnose cancer, some *real* arthritis such as rheumatoid arthritis, and a small number of structural abnormalities; but the overwhelming majority of pain continues to baffle doctors. I refer to this sea of medically undiagnosed suffering as "body and headache pain."

Q: What makes you think you know more than doctors about body and headache pain? Doctors have gone to medical school. You are just a physical therapist, so what right do you have to question them?

A: I have worked closely with all kinds of doctors for half a century. Doctors in most fields of medicine have produced remarkable advances that have earned our respect and praise. I refer to cardiac surgeons, ophthalmologists, doctors that treat cancer, and many others. Doctors that deal with body and headache pain are the exception to the rule, and their patients continue to suffer. Look at all the ads on TV for pain relievers if you don't believe me; obviously, a lot of people are still in pain.

Q: Aren't there a lot of new treatments for body and headache pain?

A: Not really. Doctors don't understand what causes body and headache pain, so they don't know how to treat it. Instead of treatment, they attempt to dull the pain with drugs. This is called *management*, not treatment. There certainly are a lot of expensive new drugs out there, but they are designed to disrupt the important alarm signal of pain that nature provided us with.

Q: You said rheumatoid arthritis is "real" arthritis. Isn't all arthritis real arthritis?

A: The term "arthritis" is meaningless today. In the old days, arthritis meant there was something wrong with a joint. Now, doctors refer to pain or stiffness anywhere in the body as arthritis whether or not a joint is involved. There *is* a joint problem with rheumatoid arthritis, but the so-called arthritis for which doctors write millions of prescriptions each year for expensive painkillers is pseudo or false arthritis. By the way, doctors have so twisted the meaning of osteoarthritis that it has conveniently become a false arthritis easily targeted by all the drug manufacturers' TV commercials.

Q: You say that doctors don't know the cause of body and headache pain. This implies there is a single cause for all body and headache pain. That's hard to swallow.

A: But it is true. It requires some background, however, to understand, and that's what my book is all about. Simply put, body and headache pain is caused by tight, contracted tissues that squeeze pain receptors.

Q: Wait a minute. Aren't there different causes for, say, migraine, carpal tunnel syndrome, and fibromyalgia?

A: If tight, contracted tissues occur in the neck and scalp, doctors call the resulting pain migraine; if in the arm and hand, carpal tunnel syndrome; and if throughout the body, fibromyalgia. The underlying cause is the same for all: tight, contracted tissues. It's really a matter of soft tissue dysfunction.

Q: How come you know all this and doctors don't?

A: My lifelong passion has been to search for the cause of body and headache pain and to develop innovative ways of treating it. My background in medical research has helped, as well as my experience as a physical therapist. But my big advantage is that I am also an artist. My creative right-brain approach has allowed me the freedom to explore new ways of doing things. Doctors are rigidly bound to concepts that don't work and are reluctant to let go and try new methods. Their arrogance hasn't helped them either.

Q: You haven't explained how it is that you know what causes body and headache pain and doctors don't.

A: Doctors do not properly examine patients who suffer pain. They look at X-rays and ask questions like, "Where does it hurt?" Doctors may press or prod here or there. That's about it. Instead of using my eyes to look at X-rays or my mouth to ask questions, I use my hands to carefully examine the body of my patient. I take as much time as necessary. The examining methods I describe in this book enable me to determine precisely where the tissues are contracted. When I use techniques that soften those contracted tissues, the pain goes away and stays away. The cause of body and headache pain is no longer a mystery.

Q: What you say seems to make sense, but then again, what about all the medical experts and specialists at those famous clinics throughout the country? They are specialists, aren't they?

A: History is replete with all kinds of respected experts and specialists who were later found to be shortsighted and downright stupid. I think of military experts who denied the possibility of air attack by the Japanese. The result was Pearl Harbor. I think of the respected French experts and their Maginot Line that caused France to lose the war. I think of respected medical specialists and how they excoriated Sister Kenny when she demonstrated humane and effective methods of treating polio patients instead of the painful plaster casts, prescribed by the specialists, that prevented recovery.

Q: I'd like to get back to your theory of tissue contraction. Why do tissues contract?

A: It's not a theory. It's something I have observed and that anyone can observe if they know what to look for and how to look for it. All living tissues have an inherent tendency to contract when irritated, from the single cell of an amoeba to the multicelled human. Tissues of our bodies contract when "insulted" or aggravated by physical or emotional trauma. The insults may be subtle and the contractions may be minute, but the effects accumulate over a lifetime, eventually resulting in significant tissue contraction.

Q: Not everyone experiences body or headache pain. This must mean that not everyone's tissues contract. Why some and not others? Also, why does one individual's neck and scalp tissues contract, causing, as you say, migraine, and another individual's entire body contracts, causing what doctors call fibromyalgia?

A: Excellent questions. Our systems are marvelously complex and difficult to comprehend. Physical and emotional insults stimulate our tissues to contract. But why some more than others and why in certain areas? In some cases, there is linkage to an activity. For example, a farmer gets painful hands from milking a lot of cows. With others, cause and effect is difficult to track. I discuss some of these dynamics in the book, but others remain to be discovered.

Q: You said that you take as much time as necessary to examine patients suffering body or headache pain. This implies that doctors do not take the "necessary time" to examine their patients. We all know how busy doctors are these days, so aren't you unfairly criticizing them? They are doing their best, aren't they? By the way, how much time do you take?

A: Doctors once assumed total care of our bodies. "If you have a problem, come to us," they said; "we know what to do." Doctors designed the present healthcare system that they imposed on us. If they are overwhelmed by so many pain sufferers, it is because they lack the knowledge to provide real treatment. The fact that there are so many pain sufferers is proof of their inadequacy. Doctors cannot wiggle out of the responsibility they assumed by saying they lack the time for proper examination. Moreover, doctors not only fail to allow enough time to properly examine their patients, they also fail to set aside enough time to properly treat their patients. I have found that two hours is necessary for a thorough hands-on examination and treatment.

Q: Two hours! You've got to be kidding. No doctor can spend two hours treating one patient. That doesn't make the slightest economic sense.

A: It makes perfect economic sense. Of course, not in the present system that doctors have hodgepodged together. In the book, I describe my vision for healthcare of the future. In the future, individuals will receive periodic "tissue checks" that start when they are young. They will be examined from head to toe for early signs of soft tissue dysfunction, before pain sets in. The two hours necessary for thorough examination and treatment will be rewarded by the prevention of all the pain that now surrounds us. Don't forget that pain is really an alarm that warns us when something is wrong with our bodies. The tight and contracted tissues that squeeze pain receptors also disturb important blood and neurologic circulation, thus causing progressive health problems. I contend that the reason the majority of individuals are now consigned to nursing homes because they are unable to care for themselves is the present inadequate system of care that has been imposed on us all.

Q: What you say makes sense, but your healthcare model is in the future. Right now, doctors don't have time to treat in the manner you describe. And if you are correct, they don't know how to treat. What are pain sufferers supposed to do now?

A: I would like to discuss briefly why I have found in my practice that a treatment session of two hours is necessary. When individuals come to me for help, I find that their problems started years earlier—often twenty, thirty years, or more earlier. Tissue dysfunction that has become established over this long a time cannot be normalized in hurried treatment sessions. All tissue systems, such as skin, fascia, muscles, and ligaments, have to be examined and treated. It takes time to do this properly. The only recourse pain sufferers have now is to treat themselves. My book describes in great detail how readers can do this using the techniques I have developed.

Q: But even those who want to treat themselves at home are unlikely to have a block of two hours available.

A: In my practice, I often treat twice a week in two hour sessions. This provides adequate treatment time per week to make inroads into an established problem. If individuals at home set aside thirty minutes each day to treat themselves, this will allow adequate time per week to normalize their tissue dysfunction.

Q: With all due respect, I don't think it is possible for people to treat themselves, no matter how much information they are given. I mean, to be treated, you have to go to an office or clinic and have someone work on you. It doesn't seem possible to reach around all over your body to treat painful areas.

A: I am living proof that it can be done. I am seventy and I am completely free of pain. However, during my life I have suffered severe pain throughout my body. For example, I suffered from severe migraines, back pain, hip pain, and knee pain. I experienced severe arm and hand pain, what doctors call carpal tunnel syndrome. I have had leg pain so severe that for an extended period I could not sleep on my right side. I once inadvertently stepped into an open posthole and painfully injured the tissues of my left ankle. Yet my body is completely pain-free and I have no physical disability. I do not have to dope myself with all the painkillers doctors prescribe for pain sufferers, *because I have no pain*. I have no pain because I successfully treated myself. Readers of this book can do the same. It takes effort and dedication, but it can be done.

As discussed in this book, doctors do not know how to examine patients for soft tissue dysfunction that may be causing body or headache pain. They are trained, however, to detect cancer and other disease processes. I urge readers to have their pain checked out by a doctor before treating their own bodies. Virginia, the state in which I practice, requires that physical therapists obtain a doctor's referral before treating a patient. I always adhere to this requirement.

Acknowledgements

Special thanks to Anna, my daughter, an intelligent, talented artist, contributor of great ideas, and an outstanding synchronized swimmer. Heartfelt thanks to Ann Longenecker for her excellent editing and wonderful support from the very start. Thanks also to Catherine Wray; she came in late to the project, but her contributions were important. Thanks to the folks at Hampton Roads Publishing Company for immediately understanding what I had to say. And a big thank-you to my good neighbor, Rick Mowbray, for telling me about Hampton Roads.

Introduction

If you suffer body or headache pain, you need to know your suffering does not have to continue and that you can be the one to help yourself to pain-free living. This book will tell you how.

I became a physical therapist almost half a century ago. In the intervening decades, I have treated hundreds of patients suffering body and headache pain, and have worked with doctors, therapists, and other health professionals in numerous work settings.

I have been involved in the study and treatment of body and headache pain for over fifty years. As a young lad growing up during World War II, I remember studying photos in *Life* magazine showing the suffering of wounded soldiers and civilians. One photo showed a wounded GI being put into a body cast. The agonized look of pain on his face spoke to me with such a strong emotional impact that I can still clearly recall it.

In 1950, I became a research assistant at the Cardiovascular/Renal Dialysis Research Laboratory, Institute for Medical Research, at Cedars of Lebanon Hospital, Los Angeles, California. That same year, I volunteered to stretch the limbs of cerebral palsy patients, thus beginning my half-century study of soft tissue dysfunction. In 1954, I was appointed supervisor of the lab and became increasingly distressed by the pain of patients suffering acute kidney disease and heart problems. This focused my interest in trying to help people escape the suffering of pain.

In 1957, I graduated from Loma Linda University's School of Physical Therapy. My experience has been in numerous areas of physical therapy and rehabilitation: staff physical therapist and supervisor in large rehabilitation centers, hospitals, extended-care facilities, nursing homes, and in-home situations; owner of a large rehabilitation and ancillary-care group; administrator of a home health agency; and a successful practice treating body and headache pain and physical dysfunction. I have worked with physical therapists, occupational therapists, athletic trainers, orthopedic surgeons, and general practitioners. My passion has been to understand the cause of body and headache pain and to develop innovative ways of treating it.

At first, I employed the techniques medical mentors taught and continue to promulgate: exercise, heat, cold, massage, ultrasound, electrostimulation, iontophoresis. However, it soon became clear to me that those modalities had only a temporary, if any, effect in alleviating pain. In fact, some caused an increase in pain. In addition, I noted early on that physical dysfunction was the constant companion of pain. Sufferers reported that their bodies were stiff, weak, and fatigued.

Doctors that dealt with pain were straight-talking in the early days of my training. When a patient with a painful and weak right arm was referred for treatment, the referral bore the simple but honest diagnosis: "painful, weak right arm." Similarly honest diagnoses were given for pain symptoms that occurred elsewhere in the body. Doctors didn't know what caused pain or physical dysfunction and they made no attempt to hide their lack of knowledge. Nowadays, doctors affix impressive-sounding diagnoses such as fibromyalgia and repetitive stress disorder onto those same symptoms. These catchy names falsely imply that present-day doctors know more about the cause of pain than their straight-talking predecessors.

Dismayed by the severe body and headache pain that was minimally affected by the treatments my coworkers and I rendered, and by the equally ineffective drug and surgical treatments doctors administered, I resolved to find more effective ways to treat pain. I intuited there must be a common underlying cause for both the pain and its ever-attendant physical problem, and that, in order for treatment to be effective and long-lasting, it would have to be directed toward that cause, whatever it was. The search for the cause continued for several years.

Then one day I inadvertently applied a more-than-usual amount of lotion to an area I was massaging. When I moved my fingers through the pool of lotion, it was as if a spotlight had been turned on! My fingertips could "see" the tissues inside. In a manner similar to the fingers of the blind discriminating the irregularities of Braille, I now was able to perceive that the painful area I had been working on was composed of tight and contracted skin, fascia, and muscle. By moving my fingers in small circles and varying the pressure, I could distinctly discern each individual tissue system. It was a moment of exciting discovery. With experience, I gained greater expertise, and I learned to use my fingers in a variety of investigative movements that provided additional important information about dysfunctioning tissues.

> *I found that wherever there was a complaint of pain there was also contracted skin, fascia, and muscle. It didn't matter if the pain occurred in the head, neck, forearm, back, or leg—it was always accompanied by contracted tissues. Areas that were not contracted were not painful.*

I found that wherever there was a complaint of pain there was also contracted skin, fascia, and muscle. It didn't matter if the pain occurred in the head, neck, forearm, back, or leg—it was always accompanied by contracted tissues. Areas that were not contracted were not painful. I also found that the only way the precise character of the underlying tissues could be revealed was by gentle exploration and the use of lotion as a discovering or "connecting" agent. The underlying cause of body and headache pain was no longer a mystery.

Now that the precise condition of the tissues that accompanied body and headache pain was identified, I explored treatment techniques that would soften and normalize those tissues. Gross massage movements were not delicate enough to be directed toward those specific tissue abnormalities my discovery agent and examining fingers disclosed. Techniques that manipulated and softened each tissue system were required. Over the next several years, I developed and refined those techniques. When they were gently applied, tight tissues softened, became normal, and the pain went away! My search for the cause of body and headache pain, wherever it occurs in the body, and real treatment of the cause, had ended in success.

I concluded that contracted tissues tightly grip and squeeze pain receptors, nerves, and blood vessels, thereby causing the symptoms of pain, fatigue, and weakness. I learned that to achieve full recovery, all tissue systems have to be examined, treated, and normalized. In the following years, I successfully treated the cause of pain throughout the body, including those types of pain with recently acquired impressive names. Patients who had been told they would have to suffer pain for the rest of their lives became pain-free and stayed pain-free because the underlying problem had been normalized. My treatments enabled patients to avoid surgery that had been ordered; others were returned to pain-free health after unsuccessful surgeries had been performed.

In addition to being a medical researcher and physical therapist, I am also an artist, primarily a sculptor. In 1986, I won a coveted position as artist-in-residence at the Roswell Museum of Art in Roswell, New Mexico. It is natural for me to use my hands as a sculptor and also as a means of examining and treating patients suffering pain. My background as a researcher and my artistic freedom enabled me to develop a treatment approach from an independent point of view, not one locked into myths, misconceptions, and erroneous notions.

All areas of the body are interrelated and interconnected, making up a continuum. Thinking of the head as being separate and apart from the neck, and the neck as being separate and apart from the shoulder, is arbitrary and misleading. Unfortunately, the conventional medical community has fallen into this fragmented concept of the human body. A problem with the knee or thigh is viewed as being separate and apart from a problem with the low back or gluteal region.

I asked my thirteen-year-old daughter, Anna, if it sounded reasonable to her that "if one part of the body is dysfunctional, then all parts of the body become dysfunctional."

She answered, "Well, if one part of the body is hurt, then the part right next to it gets affected, and then the part right next to that gets affected, then the part right next to that gets affected, and so on, until the whole body gets affected."

This leads me to offer a cautionary note about this book. When I describe problems with different "parts" of the body, it is with the understanding that these "parts" are, in reality, segments of a continuum. I have separated out these continuum segments for convenience of discussion only. It is quite different when I treat, or when other practitioners should treat, patients with body or headache pain. The next time you discuss soft tissue dysfunction with your doctor, mention Anna's theory. It might expand your doctor's horizons.

Our bodies are marvelously complex, and their workings are difficult to fathom. I make no claim to understand more than just a very tiny bit of how they function. The condition of our tissues is determined by the confluence of a great number of internal and external factors. Physical and emotional "insults" or injuries stimulate tissue dysfunction, but nutritional deficiencies, environmental and societal stressors, mental attitudes, and other factors of which I am unaware also play a part.

It is important that dysfunctioning tissues are normalized, not only to eliminate pain, but because contracted tissues squeeze vascular and neurologic structures; they interfere with the flow of normal processes, thus causing the health of the individual to become degraded. As tight, contracted tissues contribute to organ disease, I am confident that eventually everyone will be examined and treated for tissue dysfunction, because the relationship of contracted tissues and the state of one's health will be firmly established in the future.

Naturally, I was excited by my successes and attempted to share what I had learned with doctors and coworkers. To my surprise, the message of real treatment was met with a profound lack of interest.

It eventually became evident that doctors did not welcome guidance from someone outside their profession, and fellow therapists chose not to question the authority of physicians.

Sadly, patients today with body and headache pain continue to receive what they believe are treatments but in reality are merely methods that attempt to manage, that is, reduce the severity of their complaints. Until doctors understand their unseen enemy, they will joust ineffectively with its painful effects. This will continue until doctors learn how to properly examine patients experiencing body or headache pain. Currently, the doctors press on their patients' bodies with their thumbs, and this crude technique is grossly inadequate.

The medical community's attempt to deal with the secondary symptom of pain by the use of drugs, surgery, or other means without treating the underlying cause is doomed to failure, a failure that has become abundantly evident in the current epidemic of pain and suffering. The endless ads on TV touting pain relievers, including doctor-recommended ones, are constant reminders that doctors do not understand what is causing pain or how to treat it.

Doctors can find the exact cause, such as a structural abnormality, in only a small percentage of body or headache pain. The underlying cause of the vast majority of body and headache pain remains a mystery to the medical community. I contend that this mysterious cause is unidentified soft tissue dysfunction.

Therefore, after years of frustrating attempts to have doctors understand why their patients are suffering and that real treatment is available, I finally gave up on them. Instead, I decided to write a book directed not toward doctors, but toward the pain sufferers themselves. If what I write rings true, they will know they no longer have to suffer pain; they can help themselves.

Because of their ineffective focus on secondary symptoms, doctors have grown pessimistic and say what they call migraine, fibromyalgia, and chronic pain are incurable. Doctors' defeatist attitudes eclipse the truth of great hope for those who suffer body and headache pain. The cause of your pain can be treated and your body can be healed. The message of this book is that you do not have to give up; you can heal yourself of your pain.

In this book, you are given important information and detailed drawings that will enable you to locate the tissues that are causing your pain. Treatment techniques, developed over a forty-year period, that normalize the cause of pain are carefully described. Forty-eight case histories that demonstrate the success of real treatment are presented.

You will learn that tight, contracted tissues result from emotional stress turned inward, as well as from physical insults and trauma. These effects accumulate throughout the body. As they do, some areas become particularly tight, causing pain. If one of these areas happens to be the neck and head, doctors call the resulting pain migraine; if the hand and forearm, carpal tunnel syndrome; and if throughout the body, fibromyalgia.

When you finish reading this book, you will have a thorough understanding of soft tissue dysfunction, which is the primary cause of body and headache pain, and will know how you can treat yourself so your body can heal. Your pain will go away and stay away.

PART ONE:

What Causes
Your Pain?

Chapter 1

Soft Tissue Dysfunction: The Cause of Body and Headache Pain

Body and headache pain is not beamed into your body from some mysterious cloud overhead. For every complaint of pain there is an area of the body that has tight and contracted tissues. The dysfunctioning tissues press on pain receptors. Release the tight tissues, and the pain goes away and stays away.

All cells and tissues of creatures of the animal kingdom share a commonality. They are all programmed to contract as a response to being irritated. From the single-celled amoeba to the cell colony of the jellyfish to the cells that make up the tissues of mankind, cells and tissues contract when irritated. This inherent tendency of the soft tissues of our body to contract is the primary cause of our body and headache pain.

When an area of the body is insulted by injury, overuse, or by any physical or emotional stress, the tissues of that area react by going into spasm. Once tissue becomes spasmed, it stays that way—it is unable to release itself. Over time, the injured area becomes tighter and tighter, and this process may continue for days, weeks, months, or years. As time passes, spasmed tissue loses its healthy suppleness and gradually changes into thick, unhealthy tissue that constricts the blood vessels and nerves passing through it.

The dysfunctioning tissue triggers other areas of the body to become tight and contracted. The individual gradually adjusts or accommodates to what is happening to her body and is unaware how much her body has changed.

The person may have episodes or flare-ups of pain that come and go. But after a visit to her doctor and a prescription for stronger pain medication, she is, ironically, assisted to a higher level of dysfunction. Her pain may seem to go away but really does not; she merely adjusts to a new level. More time passes, more thickening happens, more pain receptors get squeezed tighter and tighter. More accommodation happens, more adjusting to having larger areas of the body affected and in pain.

After five, ten, fifteen years or more of this, extensive areas of the body have changed into thickened, scarlike tissue. Because we accommodated to them as they developed, we are unaware of them.

However, those flare-ups of pain do catch our attention, and doctors give them names. But they are, after all, merely symptoms of the underlying cause: tight, contracted tissue. Unless the underlying cause is dealt with, symptom after symptom will continually appear. Fortunately, just as every tissue has the ability to contract, the same tissue also has the potential of having the process reversed, of becoming supple and healthy and pain-free again, but only if appropriate treatment is given.

What Are Soft Tissues?

The term soft tissue can be confusing. Anatomically speaking, the body is divided into two types of tissues: hard tissues (the bones), and soft tissues (everything else).

The problem is that soft tissues can become tight and contracted, i.e., hardened. This means you can have hard "soft" tissues. The soft tissues of the body that are primarily involved with body and headache pain are:

1. skin
2. muscles
3. fascia
4. ligaments

These tissues have a strong potential of becoming severely contracted. Tendons, though frequently made out by doctors to be responsible for body pain and physical dysfunction, are rarely a cause for concern. They are tough and lie in protective sheaths that are well lubricated. Their reputation for causing body dysfunction springs from a lack of knowledge of body tissues.

Let's look at what happens to these four tissue systems that become major components of body and headache pain and physical dysfunction.

1. *Skin*. Healthy skin is soft and supple. It is easily moved over tissues that lie under it. It does not hurt when gently pressed. When skin is triggered to become dysfunctional, it tightens and thickens. It gets stuck to the tissues that lie under it. Pain is elicited when it is gently touched. The skin of the entire body may become tight and contracted, making all movements painful and difficult.

   Dysfunctioning skin is a major component of hand and finger problems. It presses down on the joints of the fingers and thumb, contributing to stiffness and pain. The skin of the palm thickens and grows taut, causing the entire hand to become stiff and unable to function properly. One sees residents of nursing homes dependent on others because of this.

   Skin overlying the area of the carpal tunnel at the base of the palm, when triggered to become dysfunctional, thickens and develops an almost plastic-like hardness, that is, becomes stuck to the fascia and ligament that form the roof of the tunnel, thus contributing to the problems there.

   An area of skin dysfunction that can have particularly serious health consequences is that of the lower extremity. Tight, contracted skin overlying the calf is frequently a component of peripheral vascular disease. The calf of someone suffering arterial insufficiency will invariably be found to have skin that is extremely hard, tight, and contracted, having an almost wooden feel. The skin is tightly adherent to the tissues underneath. This produces a tourniquet effect that squeezes arterial vessels, making their job of supplying blood to the tissues of the leg increasingly difficult. The result is not only severe pain, but tissues that are so unhealthy that ulcers develop. The tissues may become so severely damaged and life-threatening that amputation is eventually required.

If the skin anywhere on the body is thick, tight, adherent to underlying tissue or structures, and is painful to the touch, it is unhealthy and is a strong indicator that the tissues underlying it are also unhealthy. The skin and the unhealthy tissues under it need to be treated so the individual can become healthy and pain-free again.

2. *Muscles.* The purpose of skeletal muscle tissue is to shorten in length, thereby causing the joint to which it is connected to move. Healthy muscles are able to relax and lengthen again after this contractive action. When stressed, muscles progressively lose their normal ability to lengthen and remain in the contracted stage. They squeeze pain receptors, nerve endings that transmit the sensation of pain, and pain is generated. As time goes on, and they become tighter and more contracted, they become bound down by fibrotic tissue (which will be discussed in a moment).

   As years pass, the individuals feel more pain, grow weaker, and find movement difficult. They are told this is "merely something that happens with old age." This is not true. The truth is that this is what happens when a soft tissue problem is not properly treated. More than that, it is what happens when the healthcare system in place is so tragically unaware of soft tissue dysfunction that a problem that could have been easily treated years earlier is allowed to worsen and cause lifelong pain, suffering, and premature debility.

3. *Fascia.* Fascia is a type of tissue that is found throughout the body. It is a thin, strong tissue similar in appearance to Saran

Wrap, but much more pliable, and it provides protective bound-aries to the softer body tissues. Healthy fascia conforms easily to the ever-changing shapes of the soft tissues as the various parts of the body constantly move. When fascia is stimulated to become dysfunctional, it thickens, tightens, and contracts. Instead of protecting the soft tissues it surrounds, it binds them and restricts their movement.

As time passes and the fascia grows thicker and more con-tracted, the soft tissues of the body become increasingly stiff. Movement becomes painful and difficult. Yet with proper treat-ment this process can be reversed, and the thick, tight, con-tracted fascia can become soft, supple, and healthy again.

4. *Ligaments.* The joints of the body are held together by strong bands called ligaments. When ligaments are in a healthy condi-tion, they allow the joints to move freely. However, when stimu-lated to become thick and contracted, they tighten down on the joints, restricting their movement and stressing the joint struc-ture. If proper treatment is not provided and the stress is allowed to continue over an extended period, the joint may become so painfully damaged that it has to be replaced with a mechanical one.

All four tissue systems—skin, muscles, fascia, ligaments—must be examined, treated, and normalized if complete recovery is to be achieved.

The Fibrotic Fiber

So far, dysfunctioning tissue has been described as being tight and contracted. But we now have to discuss an additional and very important element of tissue dysfunction.

When the body is injured or stressed, tiny fibers appear throughout the injured area. I do not know how these fibers form or what their composition is, but I know they are there because I can feel them. I call them "fibrotic fibers" because I contend they are associated with a condition called "fibrosis," a thickening of tis-sues. My awareness of them started several years ago when I began using lotion as a discovering agent and the tiny subunits of the contracted tissue were revealed.

Since then, I have refined my perception of these fibers and realize that they coalesce to form a variety of shapes and sizes. These range from tiny hairlike configurations, to round, hard knots almost like ball bearings, to cable-like forms as thick as a thumb found in the gluteal and upper thigh areas.

When the body is injured or stressed, tiny fibers appear throughout the injured area. I call them "fibrotic fibers" because I contend they are associated with a condition called "fibrosis," a thickening of tissues. When groups of fibrotic fibers fuse, they become the thick formations one finds in advanced cases of tissue dysfunction.

The more advanced the tissue dysfunction, the greater the aggregate of fibrotic fibers. I believe these fibrotic fibers are sent out by the body to strengthen an area that is under physical or emotional stress, much as immune T cells are sent out to defend an area of the body that is under stress of infection.

When groups of fibrotic fibers fuse, they become the thick formations one finds in advanced cases of tissue dysfunction. I am speaking of the hard tissue that binds down the joints of hands and fingers; or the thick tissue of the sternomastoid muscle where it attaches behind the ear; or the plastic-like tissue overlying an unhealthy carpal tunnel.

When treating someone who has areas of thick, contracted fibrotic tissue, I find that as treatment progresses these areas of dysfunction fragment into their subcomponent forms. Finally, the individual fibers soften and disappear. The area once again is normal, healthy, and pain-free.

What Does Cumulative Trauma Feel Like?

The terms "cumulative trauma" and "repetitive stress injury" are frequently bandied about by doctors. But just what accumulates when tissues are repetitively stressed is not mentioned. I contend it is the progressive accumulation of fibrotic fibers. The greater the accumulation, the thicker the area and the more severe the symptoms.

It is difficult to precisely describe the shape and texture of fibrotic tissue, fibrotic structures, and fibrotic fibers. You have to actually feel them. Terms such as "ropy," "ball bearing-like," or "cable-like" are the best I have come up with. It is equally difficult to describe the sensations that are elicited when these areas and structures are treated and released. Expressions such as "an itchy feeling," "a feeling of release," "it feels lighter," "it feels looser," "it feels better," "a feeling like electricity" are the best my patients have come up with.

When Does Soft Tissue Dysfunction Start?

By the time a person first becomes aware that he is having body or headache pain, the development of extensive soft tissue dysfunction is well under way.

Long before the individual goes to a doctor's office and is given pain pills for backache, sinus pain, or migraines, his body has profoundly changed. As years go by and he returns for stronger medication, his body continues to change, to become increasingly tight, contracted, and fibrotic.

It is my contention that this process starts early in childhood and continues throughout the lifetime of the individual. I believe it is the result of repeated physical and emotional insults that stimulate the body to form and accumulate fibrotic tissue. I have had the opportunity to examine and treat children ten years of age or younger and have found well-developed soft tissue dysfunction in these children. Maybe "growing pains" should not be ignored after all!

The development of dysfunctioning tissue begins after any emotional or physical insult to the body. The emotional insult can result from being scolded by a parent or teacher, the stress of driving in traffic, or trouble at work with the boss. Physical insults can be from outright trauma, such as stumbling in a playground or falling out of a tree. It can take the form of postural stress, such as happens to students bending forward with heavy packs on their backs, or it can result from overuse, as happens to dancers, musicians, and computer operators.

An emotional or physical insult directed to any part of the body causes the tissues in that part to spasm. If the spasm is not treated, released, and normalized, it develops into the next stage: contraction. If this stage is not treated, it develops into fibrotic tissue.

Physical and emotional insults can be very subtle and cause only minute spasm reactions. But the results can accumulate throughout a lifetime. Thus, tissue dysfunction started in early childhood and continued throughout adolescence and young adulthood can result in profound pain and disability in later life.

In caveman days, if you were in a stressful situation—say a saber-toothed tiger was attacking you—you either ran away or grabbed a club and fought your way out of the situation. To enable your muscles to have the extra energy needed to fight or run, nature provided you with a fight-or-flight system. This system, part of the autonomic nervous system, gives you the big spurt of energy you need to pull you out of emergency situations.

In the old days, those energy chemicals were dissipated by the activity of running or fighting. Today when we are in a stressful situation, we are not afforded the opportunity of using up those chemicals. They are turned inward and cause our muscles to tighten. With each little spurt of energy chemicals released with each little stressful situation we are confronted with, our muscles and their associated tissues tighten a bit more. Over a lifetime, the accumulation of all these tightenings contributes to the tissue dysfunction that underlies your body and headache pain.

Hidden Pain

You may have lived with pain so long you don't know how much you are hurting! In order to just survive, your body has learned how to accommodate to pain, that is to say, how to block out much of your pain. We now need to discuss something I call "hidden pain."

Hidden pain occurs when your body is subjected to very slowly increasing amounts of physical or emotional stress. Let us say, for example, that the tissues of your shoulder are insulted in some manner. As a response, your shoulder tissues tighten just a "teeny-tiny" bit. This teeny-tiny bit of tightening squeezes just a teeny-tiny amount on the pain receptors located within its tissues. These pain receptors relay the teeny-tiny pain message on to your pain sensing center. (The pain sensing system is marvelously complex. For purposes of illustration, I simply call it the pain sensing center.)

The pain sensing center dismisses the teeny-tiny message of pain from your shoulder. The pain sensing center has a capability of blocking out trifling amounts of pain signals that come to it from the various parts of your body. This ability to accommodate to small levels of pain allows the pain sensing center to concentrate on more dramatic items coming to it.

You have now successfully accommodated to that teeny-tiny bit of pain. You are no longer aware of it. You no longer perceive it. But the tissues at your shoulder continue to tighten just a teeny-tiny bit more. The pain receptors are squeezed just a little bit more. Again, your pain sensing center receives the signal and easily accommodates to it. The small amount of increased pain is again blocked out.

This process of accommodating to, of blocking out messages of very small increments of pain, continues day in, day out, month in and month out, year in and year out. Although you are not consciously aware of it, you have accumulated large amounts of pain that have been stored up in the tissues of your body.

The accommodation process is not perfect. You may be aware of aches and pains here and there that come and go. When pain messages are more intense than usual, you may be aware of severe flare-ups or exacerbations of pain. Your body eventually accommodates, more or less successfully, to even these episodes, particularly if your doctor gives you pain medicine to tide you over. This is why you are not aware of how much pain there is in your body.

By the way, you are not aware of something else that has slowly been happening to your body. You have not noticed the imperceptible tightening that caused the accumulation of hidden pain. You are not aware of just how stiff and unhealthy your body has gradually become.

Hidden pain areas are difficult to describe. They need to be experienced. Here is how you may experience them: put some lotion on, say, your left forearm. Any body lotion will do for this experiment. Lotions are discussed in greater detail later in the book. Move the fingers of your right hand in slow, firm, but gentle circles on the lotioned skin of the forearm (I wish I could be there with you when you do this for the first time). Very gently squeeze the skin of your forearm just below your elbow. You will soon find areas of your skin and the tissues underneath your skin that are surprisingly painful (if this is a dysfunctioning area). In fact, you hadn't known they were painful at all.

As you explore your lotioned tissues, you will be further surprised at the variety and extent of your hidden pain areas. Some will elicit a dull, aching sensation, some will be intensely tender and painful. But all will have been hidden from your conscious awareness before you applied the lotion and performed your gentle explorations.

To sum up, hidden pain areas are components of the body's mechanism that allows us to accommodate to progressive soft tissue dysfunction. Or rather, they are a result of the body having successfully accommodated itself to prolonged periods of incremental pain and dysfunction.

TCF Relay Points

TCF ("Tight, Contracted, Fibrotic," a term I have coined) relay points are small areas of compressed tissue that relay the perception of pain to points in other areas. When a TCF relay point is pressed, pain is felt at that particular point and is also perceived at one or more distant areas.

It is interesting to note the unique pattern of TCF relay points. Just as snowflakes are different, one from the other, so are the patterns of TCF relay points from one individual to another. For example, if you press on a particular spot on one individual (say an inch below the left elbow), pain may be perceived on the back of the index finger of the left hand. If you press on the same area of another individual, pain may be felt at the shoulder, chest, or some other area of the body. TCF relay points appear to be components of the transmission system that allows one area of soft tissue dysfunction to stimulate other areas to become unhealthy.

The Five Axioms of Soft Tissue Dysfunction

First Axiom: All body tissues have a potential, a capability to contract.

Second Axiom: Soft tissue can be insulted in two ways: by physical or emotional stress, or by trauma.

Third Axiom: When soft tissue is insulted a process is started that continues inexorably onward to spasm, contraction, and fibrosis.

Spasm. In the first stage of the process, an area of the body has been insulted. The tissues of that specific area react by going into spasm. Pain receptors are squeezed, irritated, and send out signals of pain that the body accommodates to. Vascular and neurologic supply is still adequate.

Contraction. In the second stage of the process, gradually, over a few to several months, the spasmed tissues have developed into a more tightened state. Pain receptors are increasingly irritated. The body attempts to accommodate to the increased intensity of these pain signals, and hidden pain areas develop. Vascular and neurologic structures are squeezed. Other tissue areas are triggered to become spasmed and contracted. These additional areas squeeze and irritate their pain receptors, resulting in yet additional areas of tightness and pain. The problem has become "global."

Fibrosis. More time goes on and the contracted tissue becomes thicker and tougher. It takes on a scarlike consistency; fibrotic development has started. Vascular and neurologic circulation becomes strangled. There is more accommodation to increasing pain, and therefore, increasing accumulation of hidden pain areas. As the years roll on, the body becomes increasingly unhealthy and dysfunctional. Organ systems are affected; joint structures, reacting to the continued stress, become damaged; skin becomes thickened, hardened, and indurated; movement becomes difficult. The individual becomes depressed and quality of life is significantly reduced. The problem has become what the medical community calls "chronic."

Fourth Axiom: Once contracted, body tissue cannot uncontract; it cannot normalize itself.

Fifth Axiom: Just as all tissues are susceptible to a process that causes them to become contracted, so too are they susceptible to having this process reversed. With proper treatment, contracted and fibrotic tissue can once again become normal, supple, and healthy. Doctors are mistaken in their belief that when the condition has become "chronic" it is "incurable," and the sufferer must be consigned to the hopeless bin and referred to the hell of pain management centers.

Of course, the earlier the effective treatment is initiated, the more likely complete success can be achieved. However, even after tissue dysfunction has been allowed to progress and fulminate for year after year, dramatic reversals are still likely, and significant improvement in the most advanced cases is the expected outcome.

Chapter 2

Medical Treatment of Body and Headache Pain: An Overview

Doctors involved in heart and brain surgery have developed greatly improved techniques and treatments. So have cardiologists, urologists, dermatologists, ophthalmologists, and those that treat cancer. Doctors practicing in most branches of medicine have achieved results worthy of praise.

But doctors dealing with body and headache pain are the exception to the rule—their patients continue to suffer. They have only been successful in marketing themselves as practitioners deserving the respect their fellows earned, not in the treatment of their patients.

Doctors dealing with body and headache pain are good memorizers. The ability to memorize enabled them to memorize the material their teachers presented in their early schooling, thus getting high grades, which in turn got them into medical school. Being such good memorizers, these doctors memorized all the myths and misconceptions relating to body and headache pain that were written in their medical textbooks, instead of thinking things through for themselves and developing better methods of treating their patients.

Don't Throw the Patient out the Window

I had a professor of neurology who would jocularly admonish his students, "Class, study your textbooks! Study, study your textbooks! And when you are out in practice and have a patient that doesn't fit your textbook, throw the patient out the window."

Unfortunately, this is just what medical practitioners are doing when someone comes to them with body or headache pain. They have been trained to think along certain lines, to examine their patients in certain ways, to prescribe certain drugs, to perform certain surgeries. They have studied their textbooks well and continue to throw their patients out the window.

These doctors see only what they have been trained to see, and hear only what they have been trained to hear. When they diagnose someone as having carpal tunnel syndrome, they see only the wrist. They do not see all the obvious and dramatic signs of dysfunction that occur throughout the entire upper extremity. They hear only the complaints that pertain to the wrist. They do not hear the complaints of pain that occur outside that very narrow band.

The history of medical practitioners displays ample evidence of arrogant specialist mind-set. For just one example, let us look at what medical experts in Australia and the United States did to victims of polio in the 1930s. They immobilized weakened limbs in rigid and excruciatingly painful plaster casts, and arrogantly disregarded any other treatment approach. These medical specialists attacked and pilloried Sister Kenny, a nurse, when she demonstrated effective and humane treatment. It was not until thousands of victims had been tortured and denied an opportunity for recovery that these so-called experts were forced to change their ways.

So it is with the medical community of today, especially that segment dealing with body and headache pain. These self-proclaimed experts are looking in the wrong direction when their patients complain of pain. They have created a rigid concept, a rigid model. Anything that does not fit into this model is disregarded, with disastrous results for their patients.

I have tried many times over the years to get doctors to carefully touch their patients so they would understand why their patients are hurting; however, they have always been so reluctant to do so that I failed in my attempts.

Recently, I attended the neurologic exam of one of my patients. I wanted his neurologist to feel the areas I was working on. I had a tube of lotion with me and applied some to an area of tissue dysfunction.

"Feel how tight, how fibrotic this tissue is, doctor," I said, as I moved my fingers through the lotion. But the doctor declined to touch the lotioned skin of his patient. "Feel this area," I repeated, applying lotion to another area of dysfunction. Again, the doctor declined to touch his patient. This time, I took the doctor's hand and gently moved it in circular motions so his fingers could feel the fibrotic tissue. But the doctor immediately withdrew his hand and wiped off the small amount of lotion that had gotten onto his fingers. It was as if it was beneath his dignity to touch the skin of his patient.

I have done this sort of thing, from time to time, with other doctors, trying to get them to feel what I had carefully described in my reports to them about their patients. But there was always the same reaction, always the same reluctance to touch, always the fast withdrawal. I don't know why doctors are so reluctant to carefully touch their patients. Perhaps it is because of their training. Maybe they have been trained to rely on the gadgets they use to examine their patients. Doctors don't realize these gadgets give them, at best, limited information, and, at worst, false information about the cause of their patient's pain.

Take the X-ray, for example. Doctors rely heavily on this device. When someone comes to a doctor complaining of body or headache pain, the doctor will carefully study the X-ray instead of carefully studying the tissues of the pain sufferer.

What doctors don't understand is that a person can have an "excellent" X-ray, where nothing dysfunctional shows up, yet suffer severe pain. Or, on the other hand, an X-ray can look "terrible" and the person feels fine. In other words, there is no necessary relationship between an X-ray and the causative factor of a person's pain. You might discuss this with your doctor the next time he tells you that nothing showed up on your X-ray or advises an operation when something did.

It may be the doctor's training that is behind her reluctance to touch you. It may be the result of an inability to indulge in creative thinking. But even if she had been trained to do so, or had the intelligence to understand that she should do so, your doctor simply doesn't have time to carefully touch you.

I know a doctor who sees forty or more patients a day. I have been told this is not an unusually large workload. I understand that what doctors do nowadays is try to keep four or five examining rooms full at all times and to circulate back and forth as patients are cranked through, one after another. If this is so, what chance does a poor body or headache pain sufferer have for a proper examination, not to mention a proper treatment? Very little.

I have not completely given up on trying to find a doctor with whom I can discuss the relationship of pain and soft tissue dysfunction. Not too long ago, a new doctor started a practice in my area. I made an appointment to talk with him. He said he could give me a few moments. I started to describe my approach to treating painful tissue.

He interrupted. "But is it legal?" he asked. I told him of course, it's legal. He said he wasn't sure, and besides, the whole thing sounded "questionable" to him. And then he told me that he had no more time for our visit.

You Are More Than a Collection of Unrelated Anatomical Parts

When patients suffering body or headache pain visit doctors, they are not looked upon as unified beings with all parts of their bodies interconnected and interrelated. Doctors look at them, instead, as collections of unrelated anatomical parts. Accordingly, if one part hurts, its pain is thought to be separate, unique, and unrelated to the other parts.

Doctors give names to manifestations of pain. The names spring from where the pain happens to occur. If, at a particular time, pain occurs at the elbow, the doctor's attention is focused there, and the patient is told he has tennis elbow. If, at a particular time, the painful part happens to be a shoulder, attention is directed toward that part of the body, and a name is given for that pain. The name may be rotator cuff syndrome. If someone suffers from a painful head, a name is given for that painful area, and the patient is told she has migraine or tension headache.

Your body, however, is much more than a collection of unrelated body parts. All parts are interconnected and interrelated. If the tissues of one part of your body become dysfunctional, then the rest of your body reacts to that dysfunction. Pain generated by tissue dysfunction inexorably spreads throughout extensive areas of your body and will manifest itself in different parts of your body from time to time. Focusing attention on one area betrays a lack of knowledge of what is causing the pain.

Your body is much more than a collection of unrelated body parts. All parts are interconnected and interrelated. If the tissues of one part of your body become dysfunctional, then the rest of your body reacts to that dysfunction. Pain generated by tissue dysfunction inexorably spreads throughout extensive areas of your body.

Medical "treatment" of body and headache pain is directed toward attempting to reduce pain that flares up here or there as our bodies gradually tighten. Patients are given painkilling drugs or subjected to surgery directed toward a local symptom of pain. Treatment is not directed toward the underlying cause, which is allowed to worsen as the years pass. The tragic result is that countless numbers of people needlessly suffer severe and progressive pain and physical dysfunction for their entire lives.

Consider all the individuals who are forced to become residents of nursing homes because their bodies have been allowed to become so stiff and painful that they can no longer take care of themselves, and you will begin to understand the terrible toll society is paying for this medical ignorance.

Ten Approaches That Do Not Reverse and Normalize Tight, Contracted, Fibrotic Tissue

Soft tissue has a potential of contracting and becoming fibrotic. The same tissue also has the potential of having the process reversed, of becoming uncontracted, unfibrotic, of becoming healthy again if effective treatment is given. The following are what doctors currently dispense. Unfortunately, none of them will reverse or normalize contracted and fibrotic tissue.

1. *Painkillers.* Pain is our friend. At the present time, doctors consider pain to be our enemy. They should, however, think of pain as a friend, or at least an important messenger. The sensation of pain should be welcomed for what it really is: an alarm signal warning us that our bodies are becoming unhealthy. The alarm signal of pain should be promptly heeded and attended to. The focus of treatment should not be to turn off the pain signal or to somehow manage the pain signal. Instead, the focus should be to find out what is causing the signal of pain and then to fix that cause. Once the cause is fixed, the pain alarm turns off automatically.

    When we go to a dentist because of a painful tooth, the dentist does not send us to a "pain management center." She does not attempt to overwhelm the alarm signal of pain by dosing us with painkillers. If she cannot immediately find the source of the pain, she does not send us to a psychiatrist. She keeps looking for the source of pain until she finds and fixes it. The pain then goes away, because the problem causing the pain has been fixed.

    The sensation of pain is necessary for life. Occasionally, someone is born without the ability to perceive pain. The pain sensing apparatus is missing. These unfortunate individuals have a short life span. They have been denied the warning system that tells the rest of us when something is wrong with our bodies so the problem can be recognized and dealt with. We should learn from this and, in turn, should educate our doctors that the sensation of pain is important and should not be tampered with lightly without inviting dire consequences.

Put it this way: when we hear a fire alarm, we realize the alarm is our friend. We don't rush over and try to kill the fire alarm. We understand the fire alarm is trying to tell us something. Doctors should think about body and headache pain the same way the rest of us think about fire alarms. Pain is an alarm signal trying to tell them something is wrong, but it is not the problem in and of itself.

Killing the patient's alarm signal of pain with drugs or surgery without fixing the cause is medical malpractice. If we have pain of any kind anywhere in our bodies, the source, the cause of that pain, should be identified and treated.

In the old days, the doctor's answer was, "Take two aspirins and call me in the morning." At the present time, it is, "Take this expensive painkiller and come back in a month. Don't forget to pay on your way out." The next time your doctor gives you pain medication, i.e., painkillers, to block your body or headache pain, ask him if these medications are treating the cause of your pain. If the answer is yes, they are treating the cause of your pain, ask why you have to keep taking them. If the answer is no, they are not treating the cause of your pain, ask why you have to keep taking them.

2. *Exercise.* Regular exercise is necessary for the maintenance of a healthy body. I like to lift weights and perform aerobic workouts. I feel wonderful after these sessions. However, when tight, contracted, fibrotic tissues have been allowed to develop, stressing those tissues with "forced exercise" merely stimulates the formation of additional dysfunctioning tissue, thus worsening the condition.

3. *Rest.* Allowing tight, contracted tissues to "rest" (i.e., moving them very little) may give the body some time to accommodate to the pain of the tissue dysfunction, but the underlying

problem remains and symptoms will inevitably reappear in the future.

4. *Stretching*. There are two kinds of stretchings: healthy stretchings and unhealthy stretchings.

When you yawn and stretch, that is healthy stretching. A cat when it stretches—that is healthy stretching. Simply walking about, or getting up from a chair, or putting on clothing—the many hundreds of daily movements we perform, without our conscious awareness, that gently maintains tissue suppleness—these are forms of healthy stretching.

Unhealthy stretching occurs when doctors and their assistants attempt to forcibly lengthen tissues that have become contracted. Forced stretching irritates tissues that are already dysfunctional. Joint movement can be restricted by contracted skin, fascia, ligaments, and muscles. For every action there is a reaction: when force is applied to these contracted tissues, their reaction is to tighten even more. The act of forced stretching causes them to become increasingly thickened, fibrotic, and painful.

I have treated a number of individuals who participated in sports activities and regularly engaged in stretching programs that forced an increase in joint range of motion, yet these people still complained of pain throughout their bodies. Examination of their soft tissues revealed advanced fibrotic development. You might think that constant stretching would cause tissues to become supple and healthy, but this is not the case if the stretching is performed in a forced manner.

If tissues are tight and contracted, they must be gently coaxed to relax and soften; they cannot be forced to relax. Doctors do not understand this when they prescribe stretching and stretching exercise for patients. Attempting to stretch the joints of an elderly person who has accumulated the effects of years of soft tissue dysfunction is painful and unproductive, and yet is regularly performed by the medical community.

Elderly individuals frequently fall when the tissues behind

their knees get so tight that they cannot straighten them fully when they attempt to stand or walk. This condition allows their legs to buckle without warning, and down they go. The medical approach to this problem is to have therapists stretch those tight tissues. The falls continue despite the ineffective and painful stretching, and it is only a matter of time before a fall fractures an arm or leg. The tissues throughout the elderly body continue to tighten as the years pass; periodic orders to stretch the joints are given, all without result. If the aging individuals survive long enough, eventually they are unable to turn from side to side in bed and need help even to use a bedpan.

The appropriate treatment for any soft tissue problem is to soften and normalize the tight, contracted tissues. When the tight tissues of individuals who fall repeatedly after being sub- jected to years of painful stretchings are properly treated, the results are rewarding and the falls soon cease.

5. *Use of splints*. A splint prevents movement. This "forced rest" may allow the body to temporarily accommodate to an area of tissue dysfunction. However, the dysfunction remains and pain will flare up when movement is resumed.

6. *Cortisone injections*. Tissue effects of this drug are temporary and side effects can be serious.

7. *Surgery*. Cutting into dysfunctioning tissues with a sharp scalpel will not normalize them. Indeed, surgical intrusion causes scar tissue to form and may inflict damage on nerves and blood vessels, thereby complicating the problem.

8. *Muscle relaxants*. Drugs, so-called muscle relaxants included, will not normalize tissue dysfunction, in muscles or any other tissue.

9. *TENS units*. These devices attempt to block out the body's alarm signal of pain. They do not eliminate the cause of pain.

10. *Visits to psychiatrists.* Pain sufferers are grossly insulted when they are sent by doubting doctors to have their heads examined.

The Problem with Pain "Management"

The present motivation of U.S. healthcare is to maximize the efficiency of patient care, to move the patient through the system as efficiently as possible, that is, to spend as little time as possible with the patient.

This is unfortunate for the patient with headache or body pain. These problems demand appreciable amounts of time, both to investigate the cause and then to treat that cause. The pain patient gets it from both ends. The doctor is too busy to find out what is wrong, and then when the patient is sent out to the rehab center, he is moved through a conveyer-belt system consisting primarily of exercises and stretches, all designed for the practitioner to spend as little hands-on time as possible. When the insurance coverage runs out, the patient, as a sort of graduation ritual, is handed a home program of stretches and exercises, and sent on his way.

When patients do not do well, it is made out to be their fault. It is made out that they have not been diligent in doing the exercises and stretches, and therefore are responsible for the lack of improvement whereas, in reality, it is the fault of today's medical system and its practitioners.

The problem with pain management centers is revealed in their title: pain "management." The motto of pain management centers is: "Give up all hope of having the underlying cause of your body or headache pain treated, reversed, and normalized." The assumption and rationale of a pain management center is that those who enter its portals have already received appropriate, albeit unsuccessful, treatment for their pain.

In most cases, pain management centers have no intention of providing effective treatment for people suffering body or headache pain. They merely attempt to "manage" the pain as best they can so the patients can hobble around for the rest of their pain-ridden lives.

I contend there is not now a system of care that provides real treatment for those experiencing body or headache pain. If doctors knew how to treat body and headache pain, they would change their pain management centers into pain treatment centers or, better yet, pain prevention centers!

Have you made a reservation with your local nursing home? The chances are that you, a member of your family, and friends and acquaintances may end up as residents of a nursing home well before your time, because of the poor quality of the present "healthcare" system.

When I visit a nursing home, employees come to me and say, "My back (or neck or arms or legs) is killing me, what can I do?" I gently touch the area of pain and am immediately aware how tight, thick, and fibrotic the tissues are.

These are people of all ages and provide a casebook of the progressive effects of soft tissue dysfunction:

- A teenage aide with spasmed neck and back tissues hasn't been to a doctor yet; she merely complains about her pain.

- A nurse in her late twenties goes to a doctor for "pain killers"; her tissues are beginning to thicken.

- A certified nursing assistant in her forties hobbles over and shows me her terribly painful knee. I don't have to touch it. I can see the swollen tissues above and below her knee.

  She tells me her doctor has been treating it for a long time with medication and injections. A few months ago, he sent her to an orthopedic surgeon, who did arthroscopic surgery on it that made it worse. She has been going to a physical therapist for several weeks who has her doing exercises and stretches.

  "Bernard," she tells me, "it just kills me to do the things they tell me to do." She shows me how they have her bend her painful knee, and tears come to her eyes. "It hurts so bad, and it gets worse after each treatment. I'm going to stop. I can't take the pain anymore." Her doctor has recently been talking about replacing her knee with a mechanical one.

- A charge nurse in her fifties asks if I will give her back a rub. The tissues of her neck, back, and arms are noticeably thickened, and her head is stooped forward. She demonstrates a pronounced "dowager's hump" (discussed later in this book), a clear sign of significant soft tissue dysfunction. She has given up on doctors and does the best she can with over-the-counter medications.

- A woman in housekeeping says hello. I ask how her foot is doing. She says it doesn't hurt as much as it did (a surgeon removed a nerve in her foot a few months earlier), but she still gets a lot of pain. "I need to get home as soon as I can and get my feet up because of the pain and swelling," she tells me.

- The head of food service comes up to me. "Bernard," he says, "I need your advice. My whole body is getting tighter. It really worries me. I have a doctor's appointment. What will they do for me?" I look at him and see that his shoulders are pulled forward. His body from his waist up is bent forward. He walks awkwardly, with his knees pointing outward. His entire body is indeed getting tighter.

I tell them all the same thing. They need, and have needed for some time, effective one-on-one treatments directed toward the areas of their bodies that have become tight and fibrotic. They can still be helped, but there is no system of care that provides effective treatments. It saddens me to tell them this, but it is the truth. They nod their heads in agreement and tell me that what I say makes sense, and then they shuffle off to perform their various duties, pain or no pain.

Shotgun Complaints of Pain and Nerve Damage

In the conventional medical world, a patient should be cautious these days of complaining about too many areas of pain. There is a good chance she will be hustled off to a psychiatrist.

I was told by a doctor recently that physicians are trained to disbelieve the validity of claims of pain if the complainant mentions more than two or three areas of pain. This is called a "shotgun complaint of pain." The assumption is that the patient has some sort of emotional problem. This doctor disbelieved the pain complaints of a patient he had referred to me. He told me she was either neurotic or wanted a large compensation award. She had been injured in a car accident eight months earlier and since then had been complaining of severe pain in her neck, chest, both upper extremities, and her upper, mid, and lower back. Ergo, in his view, "shotgun complaint of pain." Ergo, the doctor's disbelief of the reality of her pain complaints.

What I found when I examined her was extensive areas of severely spasmed and contracted tissue. I could feel where her tissues were contracted and spasmed, and could observe her reaction when I touched those areas, so naturally I believed her pain, shotgun or no shotgun.

If doctors properly examined their patients, they would realize that what they have been calling nerve damage is in reality tight, contracted body tissues that press on nerves, thereby generating pain. The problem is with the contracted tissues. When body tissues are properly treated, pressure on nerves is released, and pain goes away.

I wanted her doctor to understand that his patient was experiencing *real* pain. So I carefully made a chart depicting the points of her complaints of pain and how they coincided with the areas of contracted tissue I could feel with my fingers. This would surely demonstrate to the doctor that his patient was experiencing real pain. But when I showed the chart to the good doctor, he looked at me as if I were crazy. I never received another referral from him. By the way, when her case went to court for a disability settlement, the doctor stated that he thought her claims of pain were not true.

When a patient complains of severe pain, her doctor may bestow upon the individual the diagnosis of "nerve damage." Frequently (may I say invariably?), this is another case of doctors not understanding their patients' bodies. If doctors properly examined their patients, they would realize that what they have been calling nerve damage is in reality tight, contracted body tissues that press on nerves, thereby generating pain. The problem is with the contracted tissues. When body tissues are properly treated, pressure on nerves is released, and pain goes away.

Doctors do not look beyond the secondary symptom of pain, which they call nerve damage. It is bad enough when doctors dope their patients in an attempt to dull the pain. The ultimate nightmare is when doctors surgically remove or permanently "deaden" stressed but viable nerve tissue, instead of normalizing the contracted tissue that is causing the problem, thus allowing the patient to become healthy again. The next time your doctor says you have "nerve damage," ask what he precisely means by that.

How Stress Affects Body and Headache Pain

There is a lot of talk these days about the painful and unhealthy effects stress has on our bodies. Because doctors do not carefully touch our bodies, they do not understand that the tissues of our bodies change in character when subjected to stress. Therefore, they are unaware that this tissue change ultimately results in pain and a lowered level of health.

For example, I think everyone appreciates that there is a connection between levels of stress and the intensity and frequency of migraine attacks. But doctors think of the relationship of stress and migraine intensity in a vague sort of way. Stress comes our way and the headache, somehow, gets worse.

What is the physical connection between the stress and the headache? Don't bother asking doctors who presently deal with body or headache pain. The cause of headaches—tight and contracted tissues—is not understood by these doctors, so what causes migraines to worsen when subjected to increased stress is also not understood.

But you, the reader of this book, now understand the mechanism that causes migraine headaches. You have learned that body tissues contract and tighten around pain receptors when subjected to physical or emotional stress. The squeezed pain receptors send out alarm signals of pain. If these happen to be located in the scalp, neck, and upper back, the resulting pain is called "migraine."

During episodes of increased stress, the pain receptors are squeezed even further, causing the migraine to become more severe and frequent. This is the connection between migraines and stress. The same dynamic holds true for any body or headache pain.

For example, patients frequently experience severe pain in their hip and thigh following hip surgery. It is reasonable to expect pain, even large amounts of pain, following complicated orthopedic procedures. However, the pain I am speaking of is very severe and interferes with rehabilitation, yet it can be effectively treated without high doses of medication.

What happens is that the surgical incision for hip surgery is invariably made through the substance of the tensor fascia lata, a thick band of fascia that extends over the hip joint down to the knee.

The purpose of this structure is to stabilize the hip and knee joints when standing and walking. Throughout the life of an individual, the tensor fascia lata is subjected to a great amount of stress as it performs its important duty. It reacts to this lifetime of stress by becoming tight, contracted, and fibrotic. When a surgeon cuts into this already dysfunctioning tissue, it severely spasms and produces large amounts of pain.

Since orthopedic doctors are not in the habit of carefully examining the soft tissues of their patients, they do not understand that the severe pain their patients experience is not due to the surgical procedure per se, but is caused instead by the hyperreaction of the tensor fascia lata.

When the unfortunate patient complains of excruciating pain and is reluctant to move his leg because of the pain, the doctor either prescribes large amounts of mind-numbing pain medication, or, more likely, exhorts the poor soul to "move through the pain." The old, inhumane and counterproductive adage, "no pain, no gain," is still, unfortunately, frequently administered.

The humane and effective approach to this painful situation is to gently palpate the tissues of the hip and thigh, so the spasmed area can be located and treated. When the spasmed tissues are softened and normalized, the pain goes away (it is surprising how comfortable the patient rapidly becomes when properly treated), and the patient begins to move his leg freely. Recovery becomes considerably more rapid.

Ironically, it is a stressed tensor fascia lata that frequently causes the hip pain and joint dysfunction that results in surgical intervention, namely, hip joint replacement. This tragically misunderstood and preventable event is discussed later in this book.

The Pain of Misdiagnosed "Obesity"

People with large bulk and heavy weight are construed to be obese; their bulk and weight is attributed to stored fat. I have treated several patients who were described by their doctors as being obese. Some were obese in the stored fat sense; others, however, were different. Their thick, heavy trunks and limbs were thickened by accretions of fibrotic tissue.

The thickened skin of these individuals, when gently palpated, was tender and painful and adherent to underlying tissues. When the underlying tissues were palpated, they also revealed themselves to be tender and painful. The tissues were thickened, not by fat, but by fibrotic tissue. The tissues surrounding the joints of these individuals were enlarged and thickened, not by accumulations of fat, but by development of fibrotic tissue.

These unfortunate individuals were doubly plagued. First, their pain and dysfunction were not appreciated, understood, or properly treated by the medical community. Second, they were described as obese and criticized for being gross overeaters.

Individuals that happen to be obese in the stored fat sense may also suffer soft tissue dysfunction. However, their doctors invariably attribute their pain to their obesity. If someone fails to lose the weight her doctor insists must be lost, the continuing pain is attributed to the continuing obesity. This is duly noted in the individual's medical record and the patient is marked down as being noncompliant (i.e., the patient is at fault, not the doctor). The truth is that the continuing pain is caused by ineffective treatment, not by the obesity.

Pain Disbelieved by Doctors

Most of the patients that come to me with complaints of body or headache pain have been disbelieved by their doctors. Many of these pain sufferers made the rounds from general practitioner, neurologist, orthopedist, psychiatrist, and back to the general practitioner. After all the medical treatments had been administered and they continued to complain of pain, their doctors had two choices:

1. They could believe their patients were really experiencing pain (which would mean they hadn't known how to properly treat them).

2. They could disbelieve their patients' complaints of pain.

Their doctors chose to disbelieve them. Suffering pain was bad enough, but what made it particularly galling for these pain sufferers was being disbelieved by the very people to whom they had gone for help.

One woman told me she hoped her doctors had found cancer. "At least they would have believed me," she said. Another woman spoke of a similar hope but this time with HIV. Both of these women and the others were relieved when I told them I believed they were having pain and pointed out the cause of their pain. They were pleased when their pain and other symptoms began to diminish, and they were elated when they became pain-free and healthy again.

The Pain Patient's Bill of Rights

I close this chapter on pain with a summary of my views that I call "The Pain Patient's Bill of Rights."

It is our right to live without body or headache pain. It is the obligation of our doctors to see that right attained and to pursue that right with diligence, enthusiasm, dedication, and intelligence.

It is our right to be believed, and to be treated with dignity and respect when we say we are having pain. We will not allow our pain to be trivialized, dismissed, or not addressed at all. We will refuse to go to psychiatrists simply because our doctors do not have the necessary intelligence or compassion to realize we really are suffering pain.

We demand that doctors acknowledge that pain is an alarm, warning us that something in our bodies is not working properly, and stop dosing us with painkillers and other nostrums designed to turn off the important alarm signal; that pain is merely a symptom, not the cause of body dysfunction; and since doctors have assumed total responsibility for the care of our bodies, that they fix the cause so the symptom of pain will go away and we will become healthy again.

It is our right to receive a thorough, intensive, and appropriate examination to determine the cause of our pain, however much examination time that may take. We will not accept one that is hurried and cursory and rushes us through as quickly as possible. It is the doctors themselves that set up the system of healthcare now in place, so they do not have the right to say they do not have the time to properly examine us.

We demand that doctors carefully examine our bodies, carefully touch our bodies so they will understand how our bodies have changed and how this change is the cause of our pain. If doctors are unwilling or unable to determine the underlying dysfunction that is causing our pain, we demand that they acknowledge their ignorance instead of pretending expertise and implying knowledge.

We will not accept the onus and responsibility for our continued pain. The inappropriate, misguided, and ineffective care our doctors have been providing should be faulted, not us.

We will strongly question the proposition that our pain is irreversible, that nothing more can be done. We understand that if we are told this, the people saying it probably do not know what is causing our pain or how to treat it.

We demand that a system of care be designed and implemented that will treat the underlying cause of our pain and diminished health, not the present one that deals only with secondary symptoms.

We, the patients suffering body or headache pain, will no longer tolerate a system that tells us to endure pain for the rest of our lives.

Chapter 3

Tissue Sculpting: Real Treatment of Body and Headache Pain

I have studied and treated soft tissue dysfunction for fifty years, and have been a sculptor for over fifty years. In my approach to treating soft tissue dysfunction, the primary cause of body and headache pain, I combine the skills I developed as a sculptor: using my fingers that shape clay to also shape body tissue, together with the discoveries gained in my half-century study of tissue dysfunction. I call this technique that I originated "Tissue Sculpting: The Art of Soft Tissue Manipulation."

In order to provide real and lasting treatment to those who suffer body or headache pain, the tissue systems of skin, fascia, muscles, and ligaments have to be carefully examined and normalized when dysfunction is found. That is to say, each tissue system has to be "manipulated." Osteopaths and chiropractors manipulate vertebrae of the spinal column. I have discovered how to manipulate soft tissue systems, and I will now pass this knowledge on to you.

Soft Tissue Manipulation Is Different from Massage

I have great respect for those who do massage. They use their hands to help their clients, and I applaud what they do, but I do different things.

I use my fingers to carefully examine and manipulate specific tissue systems. For example, I may choose during a particular treatment session to work on only the skin, or muscle tissue, or fascia, or ligaments. Perhaps in a session I may treat all those tissues, but treatment of tissue dysfunction is only effective if each tissue system is treated separately and thoroughly.

I apply my techniques directly to a specific area of tissue dysfunction and work on that particular area until it softens and becomes healthy again. If I have to work on a small area of the palm of a hand for an entire two-hour session in order to soften and heal the tissues overlying the carpal tunnel, then that is what I will do.

People who do massage are oriented to work in a more general manner, to work on the body as a whole in a particular session. And the effects they obtain can be wonderful. Clients leave their massage tables relaxed and with a sense of well-being.

Let me put it this way. From time to time, I have traded sessions with persons who do massage. I expect treating fingers to look for specific areas of tissue dysfunction, and this does not happen. True, after the session I feel relaxed overall. But I await examination and treatment if dysfunction is found, and this does not occur. Conversely, I cannot perform the broad movements they expect. My fingers continually pause in their search for specific areas of tissue dysfunction. Massage therapists are too well trained to change their habits of a lifetime.

This section presents an overview of Soft Tissue Manipulation. The following section will describe the technique in great detail, so you can treat your body or headache pain.

When I treat someone who suffers shoulder, arm, head, hand, back, or leg pain, I don't care what catchy name doctors have given that pain. It doesn't matter if he has called it migraine, carpal tunnel syndrome, or thingamabob. The treatment approach is the same wherever the cause of pain occurs:

1. Locate the dysfunctioning tissues that are squeezing pain receptors, and

2. Normalize those dysfunctioning tissues, thereby releasing the pain receptors so the pain will go away.

When my fingers find tissues that have grown tight, thick, hard, and painful, I gently apply those techniques to coax the tissues to soften and become painless.

I work with clay in much the same way. When sculpting, I gently coax the clay into the form that is in my mind. Clay cannot be forced into a different shape; it must be coaxed. So it is with body tissues: they cannot be forced into a healthier form; they too must be coaxed.

Tight, contracted, fibrotic body tissues will succumb to the gentle persuasion of a sculptor's fingers. One can be gentle and still be profoundly effective. However, treatment must be directed to specific tissue dysfunction. When this is done, the results can be astonishing.

The Connecting Agent: How to Discover the Pain's Source

In order to locate dysfunctioning tissues that squeeze pain receptors, the fingers must be intimately connected with those tissues; a connecting agent must be used. I made this important discovery several years ago.

Doctors use a connecting agent (they call it a coupling agent) when they look inside bodies with ultrasound. Without a connecting agent, gel or lotion, the ultrasound sees nothing; it is blind. Unfortunately, ultrasound cannot see soft tissue dysfunction; fingers and the connecting agent must be used for this. So it is with the fingers: they are blind to the feel of dysfunctioning tissues if they do not have a connecting agent to find the "enemy," the thick, fibrotic tissue. Invariably, the patient says, "Yes, that's just where I hurt!" Examining a patient's body without the use of a connecting agent is like the blind trying to read without the use of Braille.

In the future, when patients with body or headache pain go to practitioners for help, their practitioners will carefully examine their entire body. With the use of a connecting or discovering agent, all will be known so proper treatment can be directed to dysfunctioning tissues. When people get periodic tissue checks and treatments early on, pain and physical dysfunction will be entirely avoided.

Overview of Soft Tissue Manipulation

To reverse severe soft tissue dysfunction of long duration, treatment must include two components:

1. Enough time must be allowed for each treatment session. Soft tissue problems tend to be lifelong in development. A treatment session of ten, fifteen, or thirty minutes does not provide nearly enough time to make inroads to a problem that took thirty years to develop. I have found that it takes a minimum of two hours of continuous, uninterrupted treatment to effectively impact extensive and lifelong soft tissue dysfunction.

2. Treatment must be specifically directed toward the dysfunctioning tissue. Although soft tissue dysfunction tends to be global in nature (that is, large areas of the body are affected), the severity of the dysfunction varies from place to place, and from tissue system to tissue system (i.e., skin, muscle, fascia, ligament).

Let us say that we are treating the tissues of a painful left shoulder blade. (I selected the shoulder blade as an example of treatment because I once treated someone whose shoulder blade was crisscrossed with surgical scars inflicted in misguided and failed attempts to surgically correct a soft tissue problem.) Some areas of the skin overlying the shoulder blade are severely tight, thick, and adherent to underlying tissues. Other areas are similarly affected, but less so. Still others are not affected at all. The unhealthy areas of skin have to be located—discovered with a connecting agent—in order for them to be treated.

The same is true for the other tissue systems of that area. We need to identify dysfunctioning portions of the musculature that connect the shoulder blade to the spinal column, as well as other areas of musculature that might be involved. Dysfunctioning fascia and ligamentous tissues have to be identified so they can be treated and normalized, thereby releasing their tight hold on pain receptors.

The first step of treatment is to touch the patient's body. This simple but important act begins the process that enables the practitioner's fingers to find those tight, thick, unhealthy tissues.

We have the patient with left shoulder blade pain lying on his left side (unless this position is uncomfortable). This position approximates (brings closer together) that shoulder blade and the spinal column, thus providing some slack in the tissues and making them more easily investigated. I apply some lotion to the area of skin between the shoulder blade and the spinal column. I move my fingers in a variety of exploratory movements, up and down, in circles, and back and forth.

The first step of treatment is to touch the patient's body. This simple but important act begins the process that enables the practitioner's fingers to find those tight, thick, unhealthy tissues.

My fingers are now concentrating on the skin. They are looking for hard, thick, or lumpy areas. There's an area that's thick. I make a mental note of it and will come back later to soften and release it. As I find other areas that need treatment, I note where they are located.

The lotion is drying out, causing my fingers to drag, so I add a bit more. My fingers move smoothly over the skin again. I ripple portions of the skin gently between my thumb and fingers; this gives additional information. I find areas that become painful after a bit of gentle investigation. These are hidden pain areas and "tell" me these areas need treatment. I continue working, moving out to the shoulder blade proper.

I add a few drops of water to the lotioned skin. This provides a different connecting effect. It allows my fingers to glide over the skin just a bit differently so additional information can be elicited.

When I feel this mode of investigation has yielded an appropriate amount of information, I wipe off the lotion. I can now grasp small portions of the skin and move them over the underlying tissues. Trying small back-and-forth and circling movements, I find areas of skin that won't glide over the tissues under it because they are "stuck" to the tissues underneath. Adherent skin indicates severe dysfunction of tissues deeper in the body. So I always examine the skin carefully.

Reapplying lotion, I turn my attention to the deeper tissues, using my fingertips on the surface of the skin to gently probe and nudge the tissues underlying the skin. It is surprising how much information can be obtained this way about the condition of deep tissues. My fingers look for tight, thick musculature, fascia, and ligaments. They search for fibrotic configurations. I note anything that is not soft and supple. I ask the patient to let me know if I touch anything that is tender or painful. I note where these places are.

When I have thoroughly examined the deeper tissues, I have the patient turn onto his right side. Every examining position yields particular and unique information, although I rarely have the patient lie facedown, because this position is usually uncomfortable and tends to stretch the tissues of the back, making them difficult to palpate and treat. I explore the skin and deeper tissues from this position. Now that the shoulder is upwards, I can hold and gently move it with my left hand while with my right hand I examine the tissues that are being moved about. This gives me additional important information.

I then have the patient turn so he is lying on his back, and follow the same procedures. Gently slipping the fingers under a lotioned back in this position can yield abundant tissue information. When I have examined the skin and underlying tissues, I am ready to use the information to plan my treatment approach.

Now begins the normalizing phase of treatment. There are few things more exciting to me than locating tight, dysfunctioning body tissues that are causing severe pain, and then to release those tissues and hear the patient say that the pain is gone. Lotion, essential as a connecting or discovering agent in the examining phase, is equally important in the normalizing phase, for without it tissue manipulation cannot be directed to specific areas of tissue dysfunction.

I often start treatment by softening the skin. So, when working on that shoulder blade, I begin by applying lotion and rippling the skin bordering the spinal column at the level of the low back, and moving gently upward. All goes smoothly until I encounter one of the areas located earlier. Here, I feel the skin is thicker, so I slow down and become even gentler. At the same time, the patient reports there is pain at that spot. I try a few more rippling movements, but the thickness proves to be stubborn, so I back off and try a different method. This time, my fingers perform small, nudging movements that gently coax the stubborn area to let go. Success is achieved: The area softens, the pain goes away, and I move on.

I go back to the rippling movement. When I find other areas that are thick and painful, I pause and try to coax them to let go, to soften. With some, I am successful; with others, I will have to return at a future session when I can spend more time on them.

As treatment continues, I use a variety of movements. The greater the variety of movements used, the better the result—not only for treating the skin, but for the treatment of all tissue systems. On certain areas, I use an abundant amount of lotion; on others, a scant amount. On still others, I use water with just a bit of lotion in it. Constant variation to suit the particular situation encountered is part of the secret of success. The surprising thing is that success is usually achieved. Most of the patients I work with have been told by their doctors that they will live in pain for the rest of their lives. Their problems are extremely severe and complicated, and yet they respond well to gentle treatment, and their pain subsides.

When the skin has been appropriately dealt with, I turn my attention to the deeper tissues and structures. One of the techniques I use to release tissues lying deep within the body is difficult to describe, but I will try. Picture a loaf of bread. In the center of the loaf you have (somehow) placed a banana. Hold the loaf in both hands and gently press and release the surface of the loaf. You are creating pulsating waves that go deep and wash over the banana. So it is with the body. By gentle movements at the surface, tissues deep down can be powerfully affected.

Another technique to reach deep tissues is a variation of the nudging movement used to examine body tissues. When my fingers revisit the deep dysfunctioning tissues identified earlier, I gently nudge and coax them to relax and soften. I take as much time as necessary to do this. One cannot coax and rush at the same time.

I will use the wave variations, the nudgings, and other movements to coax the tissues of the shoulder blade and its adjacent tissues to become softened and normalized. I treat the patient while he lies on his right and left sides and faceup to gain every advantage the different approaches afford. By this time, the patient is very likely to say, "Boy, that feels a lot better!"

The degree to which you are successful in reversing tight, contracted, and fibrotic tissue and eliminating pain depends largely on two things: how severe the physical injury or emotional trauma was, and how long the time interval is between the onset of injury or trauma and when effective treatment is started.

I have treated more than one individual who was severely injured in early youth, at four or five years of age, and whose treatment, directed toward reducing and reversing the tight, contracted, fibrotic tissue, was not started until they were in their forties, fifties, sixties, or even older. In these individuals, dramatic improvement is still likely, although complete normalization is not. For others, who developed soft tissue dysfunction over their lifetime but who did not suffer severe injury or trauma, treatment is likely to achieve a near-normal result.

If treatment is started four, five, or six years following onset of the problem, then complete reversal is the probable outcome. If effective treatment is started within weeks or months of onset, before the establishment of extensive tissue dysfunction, then the expectation for complete reversal is even better. But even with the worst case scenario, significant reduction of pain and physical dysfunction can be expected.

Soft Tissue Manipulation Techniques You Can Use to Treat Yourself

You will now learn how you can treat the cause of your pain. You will get connected with your body and learn a lot about it. I think you will find it interesting and exciting. I know you will be thrilled and delighted when your pain goes away and your body becomes healthy again.

Soft tissue dysfunction underlies the pain to which doctors have affixed various names related to where in the body the dysfunction happens to occur. In the remainder of the book, I will discuss some of them and present case histories that illustrate the results of real treatment. Following each case history, I will present soft tissue manipulation techniques you can use on yourself if you have a similar problem.

Before you treat your body, a few basic ideas need to be mentioned:

1. Be focused when you treat yourself. You can't watch TV and at the same time effectively treat yourself. It takes focused attention to find those dysfunctioning tissues, and focused attention to release and normalize them.

2. The part of your body being treated must be as relaxed and comfortable as possible. For example, if you are treating your arm, rest it on a pillow; don't hold it upright.

3. The use of lotion as a connecting or discovering agent is essential for reasons mentioned earlier. Most any body lotion will suffice, although some are better than others. As you gain experience, you will develop your own preferences. I think it best to avoid those that contain large amounts of glycerin, as this makes the lotion too slippery. I have developed a lotion called Tissue Sculpture that particularly suits my approach. It develops the right amount of grip after a moment or two, in case some friction is needed. A bit more lotion, or a drop or two of water can be added, to get just the amount of slipperiness desired. Warm your lotion before treatment, if this is convenient. I have found the use of oils to be unsatisfactory.

4. Fingernails must be closely trimmed. You will be using your fingertips as well as the pads of your fingers.

5. When you work on tissue that is hard and fibrotic, it will help if you visualize it becoming soft and supple.

6. Think of what you are doing as an exciting adventure. I feel confident that when the tissues of your body respond and become healthy and pain-free, you will indeed be thrilled.

7. It may take a session or two before your fingers are able to sense the soft tissue dysfunction that underlies your body or headache pain. I gradually developed an appreciation of how tissues feel when they become tight and contracted. This book gives you the advantage of knowing what to look for before you start.

8. Keep in mind that the whole process is simple. You apply lotion to a part of your body that is painful, and your fingers look for tight, contracted tissues. You perform releasing movements, and the pain and tightness go away.

   The tissue manipulation techniques listed may look complicated at first glance, much as instructions for assembling a bookcase may appear to be complicated. But once you try them, you will find they are simple and easy to follow. Refer to the glossary for explanation of terms that are used and anatomical names and landmarks that are mentioned. I suggest that you tape-record the treatment instructions for your area of pain so you can listen to them as you do the movements.

9. I have found in my practice that a minimum of two hours each session is necessary to resolve a problem that took years to develop. There have been times when a particular pain was resolved in one session, in one hour, but those occasions were the exception to the rule.

   I frequently schedule two-hour treatments one to three times a week for the first two to three weeks, and then reduce the frequency to once a week, once every two weeks, and so on, as the problem gets resolved.

   It may be that the busy reader does not have a block of two hours available for treatment. In that case, here is my suggestion: set aside thirty minutes each day. We all have thirty minutes (although it may not seem so) to work on a serious pain/health problem. When you do this, the cumulative amount of time each week will equal or exceed the weekly amount I am able to produce in my two-hour sessions. I'll wager that once you start, you will become so absorbed with the excitement of the process that when you glance at the clock you will be amazed at how much time has flown by. Try to arrange a particular time of the day for your sessions.

10. Before you treat yourself, review the glossary to get acquainted with technique terminology. Look over the anatomical landmark drawings as well. Don't feel you have to memorize them; they are meant only to be helpful.

Soft tissue treatment is an exciting, creative experience. It is not a boring, rigid "cookbook" routine. Early on, it would be wise to closely follow treatment suggestions. However, once you gain experience, feel free to experiment if you wish. After all, every time I treat patients, I learn a bit more.

PART TWO:

How You Can Effectively Treat Your Own Pain

Glossary of Tissue Sculpting Terms

Back-and-forths: Particularly helpful in tracking and treating long, narrow bands of dysfunctioning tissue. Place one or more fingers at an area of dysfunction; move them back and forth in one-inch travels.

Circles: Thumb, single finger, or multiple fingers are used to make small or large circles. This is for exploring and treating skin or underlying tissues.

Clappings: The fingers are configured as if to clap; they are then gently brought against the tissue repetitively.

Drags: The pads of fingers or thumb are brought against unlotioned or lightly lotioned skin. This movement is similar to sweeps, but firmer, for deeper tissue.

Floats: A liberal amount of lotion is applied to the skin and diluted with a few drops of water. This allows one or more fingers to float easily over the surface of the skin. Minute patterns of fibrotic configurations can be detected in this manner. It also allows very painful areas to be treated very gently.

Jiggling: The pads of the outstretched fingers are placed against the target tissue. The distal finger joints are rapidly flexed and straightened, causing the tissues to jiggle. This gentle treatment technique creates powerful movement of large areas of tissues. It is very effective at the forearm and calves.

Kneading: The movement is the same as kneading bread or pastry.

Nudging: This technique is used to normalize well-defined areas of tissue dysfunction, and thumb or fingers can be used. Approach the border of the target tissue and direct the movement toward its center. Imagine a raisin glued to a tabletop. You want to soften that raisin as much as possible, so you gently and patiently nudge it from all directions.

Palming: The palm is placed closely against the skin of the target area and moved in circles or back-and-forths. This technique is frequently used on unlotioned skin as a means of loosening adherent bonds.

Pincering: The thumb and forefinger are placed at opposite sides of the target tissue. For example, the thumb is placed on the palm of the hand, and the forefinger on the top of the hand. Circles, push-pulls, and back-and-forths are frequently used movement patterns. This can be used on joints, skin, or deep tissues.

Probes: The tip of a single finger is used to explore deeper tissues.

Push-pulls: This is one of the movements of pincering. The tissue is between the thumb and forefinger. The thumb pushes the tissue against the forefinger, the forefinger then pushes the tissue back against the thumb so that the tissue is pushed and pulled.

Shaking: This can be used at a joint or with a broad area of tissue. Pincer the joint or tissue between the thumb and forefinger, and gently shake. This movement is particularly useful with tissue configurations such as the biceps, or with joints such as at the base of the thumb.

Skin Grasping: This is used to free a local area of adherent skin from underlying tissues. Grasp a small bit of skin between thumb and forefinger; move it in small circles and back-and forths.

Skin Rippling: This technique is used to identify and normalize (1) thickened, fibrotic areas of the skin, (2) hidden pain areas, and (3) areas of the skin that are adherent to underlying tissue. Place thumb and fingers on the skin; move the thumb toward fingers. As this is performed, allow the skin to move wavelike under the advancing thumb. Thick, adherent skin will not ripple.

Slapping: Here, outstretched fingers very gently slap broad areas of tissues, setting up waves. Slapping is frequently used as a finishing technique.

Stationary Pressing: A single finger, multiple fingers, or the thumb can be used to press gently but firmly on a tissue area. This is useful for treating severely painful areas, where movement would be uncomfortable, and it's useful in softening creases.

Sweeps: The flat edge of the thumb, single finger, or multiple fingers are used in sweeping motions, as if you were smoothing down the hair of your forearm, or brushing crumbs off a tabletop. This is useful for gently treating the skin.

Tapping: One or more fingertips set up local waves in underlying tissues.

Waves: Here, wavelike patterns go down into deep tissues. These are set up at the surface of the body by gentle pulsating movements of the palms or finger pads.

Anatomical Landmarks for Tissue Sculpting

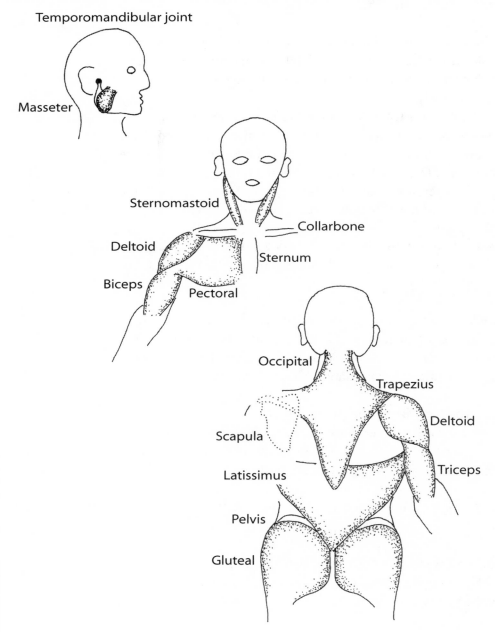

Temporomandibular joint

Masseter

Sternomastoid

Collarbone

Deltoid

Sternum

Biceps

Pectoral

Occipital

Trapezius

Deltoid

Scapula

Triceps

Latissimus

Pelvis

Gluteal

Arthritis

The word "arthritis" has lost almost all meaning these days. In the old days, arthritis meant an inflamed joint ("arthro" = joint, "itis" = inflammation). Doctors have so twisted the meaning of the word that nowadays this is no longer true.

We are told by doctors that osteoarthritis is the most common form of arthritis, and we are constantly bombarded by TV and magazine commercials hawking the multitude of osteoarthritis painkillers: "Oh, the terrible pain of osteoarthritis."

Doctors tell us that osteoarthritis is caused by wear and tear of the joints. But wear and tear of joint tissues is a benign process that occurs slowly without inflammation and rarely is accompanied by pain. This is not arthritis. The proper term for this benign process is arthrosis. There is no need to take all those expensive and potentially harmful, doctor-recommended painkilling anti-inflammatories for this condition. In fact, prolonged use of these drugs may actually damage bone and cartilage.

By the way, inflammation is a normal healing process that should not be tampered with lightly. Instead, the cause of inflammation should be determined and dealt with.

Doctors do not know how to examine patients suffering body or headache pain. They therefore do not realize the pain and stiffness affecting so many millions, that they have been calling osteoarthritis, is really soft tissue dysfunction occurring outside innocent joints.

Of course, some doctors are more creative in the names they invent for so-called arthritis. Take the following case, for example.

Case History

A printer who heard of my work had obtained a prescription from his physician and arranged for an appointment. He had been treated for several years by an arthritis specialist for what the specialist called "serum negative arthritis." The printer suffered severe pain throughout his body. The pain was constant with episodes of exacerbated, unbearable pain.

The problem had started seventeen years earlier after he injured his back in a fall. Gradually, over the years, the pain spread from his back to all parts of his body, including his arms and legs. The arthritis specialist had treated him with various medications and painkillers, but his symptoms had steadily worsened, and the frequency and intensity of the flare-ups had recently increased.

At the time of our first treatment, the pain in his hands was so severe that he could only use them as "paddles," with fingers outstretched. He was greatly concerned that, because of his inability to use his hands properly, he was about to lose his job.

When I palpated his body, I found that all of his tissues were tight, contracted, and extremely painful, from the top of his scalp to the soles of his feet. But at the end of the first treatment, he stated that his pain was down seventy-five percent. He could use his hands in a near-normal fashion. He was delighted.

I continued to work with him for two months. He was then free of any pain and could perform his job without any problem.

He called a few months later to report a flare-up of pain, and returned for a few more treatments. The flare-up coincided with a stressful marital problem. I continued to see him every three or four months for flare-ups that coincided with marital-stress episodes. These flare-ups responded favorably to one to three treatments.

Two years after I had first seen him, he called to say that he and his wife had separated and that he was leaving the area. He thanked me for the help I had given him and said he was feeling fine.

This person had suffered severe pain and physical dysfunction for several years because of the inability of his doctor to understand what his problem was and how to properly treat it. He had been given various arthritis and pain medications, all to no avail.

We found, however, that his pain was caused by tight, contracted tissues that squeezed pain receptors. When I released the contracted tissues surrounding his pain receptors, his pain went away. During the episodes of marital stress, his body tissues retightened, again squeezing the pain receptors located within them.

The tissue systems of our body, primarily the skin, muscles, fascia, and ligaments, respond to physical and emotional insults by contracting. In other words, both emotional and physical stress can cause soft tissue dysfunction that results in pain.

As mentioned earlier in this book, the tissue systems of our body, primarily the skin, muscles, fascia, and ligaments, respond to physical and emotional insults by contracting. In other words, both emotional and physical stress can cause soft tissue dysfunction that results in pain. Emotional stress was an important factor of this individual's soft tissue pain that was misdiagnosed as arthritis pain.

Soft Tissue Manipulation Techniques

Soft tissue dysfunction that is misdiagnosed as arthritis can occur anywhere on your body. I suggest you start by examining and treating your arms, hips, and knees. Refer to "Carpal Tunnel Syndrome," "Hip Pain and Degenerative Joint Disease," and "Knee Pain" for soft tissue manipulation techniques.

Back Pain

X-rays, MRIs, and CAT scans identify the cause of only a small percentage of back pain. Did you know that over 80 percent of back pain remains unaccounted for by doctors? They will continue to be baffled by back pain until they begin to carefully touch their patients.

I have observed all kinds of medical treatments that are directed toward back pain, going back fifty years to when I was a research assistant at Cedars of Lebanon Hospital in Los Angeles in 1950. I have studied the consequences of mutilating surgeries, as well as the poor results of traction devices, medications, and modalities such as exercise, stretches, and ultrasound.

Over the years, numerous medical innovations, some of them so-called high tech, have been introduced. In one large facility, I saw physical therapists tightly strap sufferers of severe back pain into cages controlled by computers. The victims were exhorted to push, bend, and twist their painful backs with all their might against the force of their computer-driven cages. If they refused or did not push mightily enough, no matter how severe the pain, negative notations were entered into their charts, and they were branded as malingerers.

Case History 1

A young woman was referred to me because she had been experiencing severe back pain that had been progressing over a period of two years. At first, the pain had been mild and intermittent, but as the months went by, the pain had become increasingly severe and constant. She had been given muscle relaxants, pain medication, and stretching exercises, but the pain continued to worsen.

When I examined her, I found that the tissues of her middle to lower back were tight and contracted, and in addition the tissues of her right gluteal area were tight, contracted, fibrotic, and painful to mild palpation. At first, she responded rapidly to treatment. Within two weeks, she had minimal, infrequent pain. But then her improvement slowed. I continued to treat her twice a week for one month, but her remaining pain stubbornly resisted treatment.

At that point, I found something interesting: a small, hard "knot" of tissue in her right gluteal area. I concentrated my efforts on reducing the knot and, as it softened, her remaining pain rapidly cleared.

Just before she was discharged from treatment, she recalled that she had been given a penicillin injection in exactly that spot a month or two before she began experiencing her back pain. Apparently, the penicillin had irritated the tissue at the injection site, causing it to spasm, contract, and become fibrotic. Gradually this area had triggered other areas to contract and become painful. The result eventually was the severe and continuous pain she was experiencing when she came for treatment.

It is highly unlikely that the sequence of events that led to this woman's back pain would have been unraveled unless someone had taken the time to carefully examine and treat her. She would have been added to the millions who suffer severe pain for the entirety of their lives when they don't have to.

Case History 2

A patient was referred because of back pain that had persisted and progressed over a thirty-year period. He had injured his back in his teens when he attempted to lift a heavy weight.

At the time of the injury, he experienced severe, painful spasm of his low back. Pain radiated down both legs. His doctor admitted him to a hospital, where he was placed in continuous traction and was given strong pain medication. Following his discharge from the hospital, his symptoms gradually eased, but he was "never the same" after this.

From time to time, he had flare-ups of pain of varying intensity. He could go for weeks or months with little or no pain, but was always aware that his low back was his problem area and that if he was not extremely careful, the pain in his back would flare up intensely. Or he might go for long periods of time with little or no pain, when for no reason he would have a flare-up of severe, excruciating pain, accompanied by intense spasming and tightening of the tissues of his lower back, incapacitating him for one or two weeks. He was given anti-inflammatory medication, muscle relaxants, and pain medication when these flare-ups occurred, which helped to take the edge off the severity of pain.

As the years passed, he noticed that the episodes of pain were becoming more frequent and intense and were lasting longer. By the time he came to see me, his life had become one long, continuous misery.

When I examined him, I found that the tissues of his entire back, particularly from his middle to lower back, down to his gluteals, were tight, contracted, and severely fibrotic, and very tender to light palpation. Thick, tough, fibrotic bands around the brim of his pelvis were easily palpated. The skin overlying these areas was thick, adherent to substructures, and was very tender to light palpation.

The severity of his pain began to subside early in treatment. However, the thick, fibrotic tissues were slow to respond. By the end of three months of treatment, he was free of pain, although appreciable amounts of the thick, fibrotic bands that had developed over the years remained.

Occasionally, he felt that his back was retightening. At those times, he called for an appointment, and we resoftened the tissues that had begun to tighten again. I kept him pain-free over a four-year period, but after that I lost track of him.

Soft Tissue Manipulation Techniques

Soft tissue dysfunction of the upper, middle, and lower back, as well as tissues of the gluteal region, can contribute to back pain. All these areas will require investigation and possible treatment. It will be challenging for you to treat those areas, but it can be done.

Of course, other tissue areas may also contribute to back pain—the lower extremities, for example. Indeed, the entire body is a continuum. As stated earlier, I have separated out the different body "parts" for convenience of discussion only.

Treat yourself while you lie on your side, first one side, then the other. Lying facedown stretches the tissues of the back and makes it difficult to work on them. I suggest that you lie on a sofa with your back facing the back of the sofa, but a few inches away from it. This allows you to lean the elbow of your treating hand against the sofa during treatment, thereby reducing fatigue and providing leverage.

Dysfunctional areas that cause low back, hip, and sciatic pain

Place a pillow between your legs. This will not only make your knees more comfortable, but, even more importantly, will put some slack in the uppermost gluteal tissues, making their treatment more effective. I suggest that you cover the sofa with a sheet and some towels, the chances are that some lotion will drip on them. Have your warmed lotion and a cup of warm water close by.

This first treatment will be a "get acquainted with your body" session. Relax, you have a lot of work ahead of you. Pace yourself; don't try to get it done all at once.

Let's say that you are lying first on your left side. Reach back with your right hand and run it over your back and gluteal areas.

Do this first without lotion, just to get a preliminary feel of things. Reach up as high as you can in the direction of your head. Go down to the gluteal area. Bend your knees toward your chest and see how that stretches the gluteal tissues. This makes it difficult to treat them. You will treat the gluteal tissues with your knees straight.

Apply some lotion to your back. Start up as high as you can reach. With multiple-finger back-and-forths, follow the muscles that run along the side of your backbone. Use the knuckles of your fingers, then the pads of your outstretched fingers. Alternate this throughout the treatment to avoid fatigue.

Go down as far as your pelvis. While you are down there, preliminarily explore the rim of your pelvis with thumb circles and back-and-forths. Look for fibrotic thickenings that are adherent to your pelvis; these will require your future attention.

Concentrate for the moment with the muscle group that lies parallel to your spinal column. Get acquainted with it. Pincer it and perform push-pulls. Is it stiff and adherent to the spinal column? Perform finger sweeps. Do you find painful, hard, fibrotic thickenings? How about the overlying skin? Is it thick and adherent? Explore the spinal column. Can you feel the contour of each vertebrae, or is the spinal column covered with thick, cartilaginous tissue? This will require extensive treatment to reduce.

Follow your spinal column down to your tailbone. Do you find thick and painful bands of cartilaginous tissue covering the bones of that area? If so, these will require patient, extensive treatment using thumb and finger circles, back-and-forths, and nudges.

Now explore the gluteal tissue. Straighten your knees to put some slack in those tissues. How does the skin feel? Try ripples. Any thick and adherent areas? What about the deeper tissues? Try thumb and multiple-finger circles and probes. Try jiggles and kneadings. Try pincering with back-and-forths. Look for tight, thick, painful bands. In the gluteal region, these can be as thick as your thumb.

The Abdominal Band

When there is a soft tissue dysfunction of the lower back, fibrotic tissue may over time spread out from the central area of the spinal column to the abdomen. I call this expansion of fibrotic tissue the "abdominal band." Eventually, the fibrotic tissue becomes extensive and adheres to the contents of the abdominal cavity.

I suspect this adherent, space-occupying tissue plays a significant role in degrading the health of the organ system. I feel certain health practitioners of the future will understand considerably more about the relationship of this space-occupying, adherent fibrotic tissue and organ health than is presently known.

I do know that patients I have treated for low back problems have frequently complained of severe constipation. When I find, treat, and normalize the band of abdominal fibrotic tissue, the symptoms of constipation gradually recede. I have also found that there is a relationship, at times, between abdominal fibrotic tissue and symptoms of hiatal hernia in the area above the stomach.

If there is a relationship between abdominal fibrotic tissue and these more observable symptoms, what relationships might well exist with more subtle organ system problems that lead eventually to a lowered level of health?

I do not recommend that laypersons treat the abdominal area, but that you should consult practitioners who are properly trained in this.

> *Patients I have treated for low back problems have frequently complained of severe constipation. When I find, treat, and normalize the band of abdominal fibrotic tissue, the symptoms of constipation gradually recede. There is a relationship, at times, between abdominal fibrotic tissue and symptoms of hiatal hernia in the area above the stomach.*

Breast Pain

Tight, contracted tissue of the breast can cause severe pain. This problem usually responds quickly to soft tissue manipulation.

Case History

A woman in her forties was referred to me for treatment of severe and constant pain of her left breast. She had suffered the agonizing pain for nine years and was convinced that cancer was the only thing that could cause such excruciating pain, although three mammograms were negative. For those nine years, she had been treated by doctors with pain medication and anti-inflammatory medications. But during all those years, her pain had grown increasingly more severe, more unbearable. Finally, a nurse practitioner who knew of my work obtained a prescription allowing me to treat.

Palpation revealed thick, contracted tissue running from her left pectoral area down into her entire left breast. After a few minutes of treatment, as her tissues softened and her pain eased, she told me that at last she realized that she did not have cancer.

She responded well to treatment and was discharged after four treatments, pain- and symptom-free.

Soft Tissue Manipulation Techniques

All possibility of underlying organic problems such as cancer must be ruled out. Then lie with your upper body propped up with pillows or a bolster. Apply lotion up around your collarbone. Treat the skin first, with ripples and thumb sweeps. Let your fingers look for areas of skin that are painful, thick, and adherent to underlying tissues. When found, release them with nudges and gentle single-finger probes. Work over the entire breast.

Support the breast upwards with one hand, and with the other make single-finger and multiple-finger sweeps along the bottom of the breast. Pay particular attention to this area, especially if your breast is large and heavy. Use plenty of lotion. The tissues here can become surprisingly thick, hard, and painful.

Go back up to the collarbone area and explore the underlying tissues with multiple-finger circles, back-and-forths, thumb sweeps, and kneadings. You are likely to find excruciatingly painful areas up where your collarbone meets your shoulder joint. Hidden pain can radiate from here down into your breast. Work down into the rest of your breast with similar maneuvers. Treat with the breast supported with your other hand, and also with it unsupported, for the greatest variety of treatment effects. Finish each treatment with waves.

Bunions

Bunions are the tip of an extensive iceberg of soft tissue dysfunction. If the tissues of someone suffering this bony misalignment are carefully examined, contracted skin, fascia, muscles, and ligaments will be found in the foot, leg, thigh, and probably in the low back. Indeed, tissue dysfunction throughout the entire body is likely.

When one part of the body becomes dysfunctional, the rest of the body responds to that dysfunction. This analysis holds true for soft tissue dysfunction associated with bunions.

Doctors tell us that ill-fitting shoes cause bunions. However, a shoe does not have the magical power necessary to beckon a bunion to spring forth. The cause is tight, contracted tissues that *pull* bones out of line. Shoes can contribute to the problem, but tissue tightness does the job. The humane approach here is to prevent bunions from forming by early soft tissue treatment. If bones have already been pulled out of alignment, then the tight tissues should be softened and normalized, thereby allowing the bones to go back into place.

Case History

A woman called and asked if I could help her "bunion problem." She told me she was in her early fifties and that for several years the bunion on her right foot had become increasingly painful. The problem started in a small area that hurt when it rubbed against her shoe.

The pain was now excruciating. She was aware of an ache and tightness when she awoke in the morning, and unbearable pain when she put on a shoe or took a step. Her doctor told her she needed surgery, but she declined this because of the horror stories she had heard about foot surgery.

When I examined her, I noted that the great toe of her right foot was pulled out of alignment, causing the tip of the toe to be drawn under the adjacent toe and the base of the toe to form an infamous bunion.

The tissues attached to the base of her great toe were thickened and extremely painful to the lightest touch. Severe pain was elicited when I gently attempted to realign the toe. The skin overlying the area was hard and plastic-like and was adherent to underlying tissues.

When I palpated the rest of her foot, I found that all the tissues were tight and thick. I discovered hidden pain areas throughout her foot and up into her calf. She was surprised by all the severe pain she had been unaware of. The tissues of her left foot were also tight and thick, and the great toe was slightly misaligned. She said she was having some pain there, but nothing like the other foot. As we chatted, I learned that she suffered from headaches, sinus pain, tight and painful arms and legs, and her neck and back hurt. Here was another case of global dysfunction.

I spent the two hours of the first treatment on her right foot. I treated the entire foot but concentrated on the skin and underlying tissues surrounding her great toe. By the end of the session, she was able to wear her shoe and bear weight with "very little" pain. She was pleased and encouraged by the results of just one treatment.

When she arrived for her second treatment, she reported that her bunion was much improved. She had not experienced the usual morning ache and tightness, and the pain of walking was less. I again concentrated on the tissues surrounding her right great toe, but spent an increasing amount of time on the rest of her foot. By the end of the treatment, the skin overlying the base of the toe was soft and supple and moved easily over the underlying tissues. I could manually align her toe to a normal position without producing any pain, although it had a tendency to drift back to its old misaligned position.

I suggested that she continue treating her foot between sessions in the manner she had observed so as to speed up recovery. I was able to spend a few minutes on her left foot. Although she was aware of little overt pain, we did find considerable hidden pain.

When she reported for her third treatment a week later, she said that she was extremely pleased with her progress. Her toe remained in proper alignment and she no longer had any pain. I extended treatment to her calves. I continued treatment at decreasing frequency for the next two months. At the end of this time, the tissues of both feet and legs were soft and supple, she had no pain, and her toes were properly aligned.

Soft Tissue Manipulation Techniques

Tissues of your entire lower extremity need to be examined and normalized. However, if you already have a painful bunion, you want to get relief as soon as possible, so let's start work directly on that bunion. We'll assume your right foot has the bunion. Have lotion (warmed, if convenient) and a cup of warm water standing by.

Cross your legs so your right foot is resting on your left knee. Apply lotion to the hard, crinkly, and tender skin overlying the bunion. Examine the skin with thumb and fingers. Notice how stiff and adherent to underlying tissues it has become; it is almost as hard as plastic. You will be surprised how quickly it will soften and become healthy once again.

Use the forefinger of your left hand and the thumb of your right hand. Gently ripple the skin toward you with your finger and away from you with your thumb. Nudge it and coax with circles. Add a few drops of water to make the lotion a bit more slippery, and gently work on the skin. Take your time. Your gentle coaxing is already beginning to soften and free it from the tissues underneath.

Move down to your instep, using both your thumbs to perform circles and nudges. Sweep with the thumb of your right hand.

Notice all the tight, contracted tissues underneath. Work back to your heel. Perform thumb sweeps along the length of your foot, from heel to bunion. Observe how your great toe moves side to side. You are now working on primary tissues that pulled your bones out of alignment. Treat thoroughly with thumb circles and nudges. I am sure you are finding painful, contracted tissues. Be glad that you are, because you are discovering and treating the cause of your bunion. This is your first treatment, a get-acquainted session, so it is time to move on.

Apply lotion to your heel and continue with thumb circles and sweeps. Work the heel thoroughly. Your entire body weight has pounded it daily, every time you have taken a step. Look for tight, painful areas; they will respond and soften.

Return to the bunion area. Extend treatment to the ball of your foot. Circle and nudge with both thumbs. Work the joints with push-pulls. You are beginning to loosen the joints of your foot. Stiff joints guarantee an unhealthy foot. The joints of the hand should be soft and supple; so too should be the joints of the foot. Examine and treat the joints of your toes. Move down to the joints of the arch of your foot. Loosen them with push-pulls. You will be surprised how quickly the joints of your foot will respond to gentle treatment. Your foot is rapidly becoming healthy and pain-free.

Place your thumbs on the sole of your foot and examine the skin and other tissues on the top side of your foot with your fingers. You will likely find very painful areas at the base of your toes. They also need to be softened and normalized.

You have now treated the primary areas of your foot that caused your painful bunion to form. Additional gentle treatments will further soften contracted tissues, enabling misaligned bones to go back into their proper positions. Your foot will become pain-free and healthy. Isn't that a lot better than having doctors violate the tissues of your foot with scalpels, forceps, and bone cutters? If you want to *avoid* bunion formation, and at the same time ensure pain-free, healthy feet, perform the above procedure from time to time.

Other areas of foot pain that doctors have given impressive sounding names, such as plantar fasciitis and Mortons's toe, will also respond to the preceding soft tissue manipulation techniques.

Bursitis

The term "bursitis" is vague and misleading. It is commonly misused by doctors as a diagnosis of convenience, much as the diagnosis of arthritis is frequently misused. The purpose is to put a name, any name, on an area of pain.

Some joints of the body are contained within a sac. Frequently, when someone complains of pain perceived to be coming from a joint, this sac, or bursa, is blamed as the culprit. This is rarely the case. The cause of pain is usually tight, contracted body tissues outside the joint.

Case History

A gentleman in his early sixties was referred to me with a diagnosis of "bursitis of the right hip." He had developed pain in a small area of his hip over a six-month period which had progressively worsened, and it was now severe and constant. He received anti-inflammatory medication and an injection of cortisone, without any reduction of symptoms.

When I palpated the tissues of his hip and thigh, I found tight, contracted, fibrotic tissues from his hip down to his knee. I worked on those tight tissues for two hours. When the gentleman got up and walked about, he no longer experienced any pain.

When he returned for further treatment two days later, some pain had returned, although not to the level of the first treatment. I continued to treat twice a week for six weeks. At the end of that time, the contracted tissue throughout the treated area was softened and supple, and he was discharged, pain- and symptom-free.

What had been diagnosed as bursitis was a symptom of pain perceived at his hip but caused by contracted tissue throughout his lower extremity.

Soft Tissue Manipulation Techniques

Soft tissue dysfunction causing the misdiagnosis of bursitis can occur at areas throughout the body. Joints frequently misdiagnosed as having bursitis are those of the shoulder, hip, and knee. Refer to "Carpal Tunnel Syndrome," "Hip Pain and Degenerative Joint Disease," and "Knee Pain" for soft tissue manipulation techniques.

Cancer

Soft tissue dysfunction frequently underlies body and headache pain. Of course, there are other causes of pain, such as cancer. However, pain generated by soft tissue dysfunction may coexist with organic pain, and may even be the primary pain contributor. Because of the ignorance of their doctors, many patients suffer needlessly because the soft tissue component of their pain is not addressed. While I do not treat cancer, the following case provides an interesting look at the pain and cancer connection.

Case History

I was successfully treating a woman for a shoulder problem, and she was pleased with her rapid progress. At her second treatment, she said that since I had been so successful in treating her painful shoulder, could I help her sister-in-law?

She went on to tell me that her sister-in-law was suffering from advanced bone cancer. She had just returned home from a hospital, and was being cared for by a hospice group. The bone cancer had advanced to such a point that her sister-in-law was suffering continuous, excruciating pain in her lower back, which increased significantly with the slightest movement. The pain was uncontrolled by medication except at levels that caused her to become lethargic and unresponsive. Not only was her sister-in-law suffering, but her pain was causing anguish for her husband and other loved ones. My patient asked if I could help.

I said, no, I couldn't help cancer pain, that I treated soft tissue dysfunction and pain associated with soft tissue dysfunction. Pain caused by bone cancer was something I couldn't help. But she persisted, saying they had tried everything else, and her sister-in-law was still suffering; they couldn't turn her in bed without her crying out in pain, and could I please go and see if there was *anything* I could do to ease her pain. Reluctantly, I told her I would call the hospice group, and see if they would get me a doctor's order to treat, but I was doubtful I could do anything.

The hospice group got the order for me, and that evening I went, although with great trepidation. I took a microcurrent unit, thinking this electronic device was the only thing that might have a chance of easing the woman's pain. I found the sister-in-law lying in bed on her back, grim-faced with pain. Her family was gathered around her. I told them the unit I had brought with me *might* be able to help.

I carefully reached under her to place the electrodes. To my surprise, I found tight, contracted, and fibrotic tissue in her low back. As I gently touched the area, I asked if that was where she was hurting. She said yes.

Instead of using the microcurrent, I applied some lotion and proceeded to gently work on the contracted tissue. After forty minutes, I felt the tissues soften, and I asked if she could move. To her surprise and joy, she moved easily with very slight discomfort. She was able to sit up without pain. She and her family were delighted.

I told them I would not be able to come back on a regular basis and that it was likely the area would tighten again, at least to some extent. I reassured them that I would show the hospice group what I had done so they could continue the treatment if necessary.

The next day, I called the hospice group and told them what I had done and that I would be glad to demonstrate the treatment. The nurse on the phone sounded skeptical that I had been able to help a "bone-cancer pain" with "massage." At the very least, she was not interested enough to take me up on my offer to show her and the other nurses what I had done. I had discharged my patient after her second visit and didn't hear again from her, her sister-in-law, or the hospice group.

The doctors and nurses had confused the severe pain caused by contracted soft tissue squeezing pain receptors with the assumption the pain was caused by the bone cancer.

If a doctor happens to read this, perhaps now she will realize why some patients complain of pain so severe they think they have cancer, and yet nothing shows up on their X-ray or other tests. If the doctor carefully touches the tissues of these patients, she will begin to understand why they are hurting so much.

I have had little experience in treating individuals who have cancer, and those were in a rehabilitation setting, not for the treatment of pain they might have been experiencing. The above case history is the one exception. It may well be that pain of soft tissue origin is confused with the pain caused by cancer in other individuals. I suspect this happens, but because of my lack of experience in this realm, I cannot suggest particular areas to be examined. Refer to the section that corresponds to where your pain is occurring and see if you find tissue dysfunction there that lessens when you apply soft tissue manipulation techniques. But before you treat, discuss this with your oncologist; there may be medical reasons that tissue manipulation should not be performed.

If, for any reason, you choose not to perform tissue manipulation with the intent of reversing dysfunction, the gentle techniques of sweeps and floats will provide a gentle, soothing effect. This might be an occasion for you to relax and let a friend or loved one apply warm lotion with a loving touch.

Carpal Tunnel Syndrome (or Repetitive Motion Disorder)

We know that carpal tunnel syndrome, the terror of computer operators and many others, is caused by repetitive motion of the wrist and that the "best" treatment for carpal tunnel syndrome is the use of wrist splints, rest, exercise, and the injection of cortisone into the wrist. If these procedures fail, surgery will be necessary, and if one surgery is not successful, then additional surgeries will have to be performed. If carpal tunnel syndrome has become too severe, the condition is "irreversible"; even surgery cannot help. If you have any doubt about the accuracy of these statements, ask any doctor.

False Notions about Carpal Tunnel Syndrome

The above statements reflect false notions doctors have about what they call carpal tunnel syndrome. Doctors produce a diagnosis of carpal tunnel syndrome by provocative testing of the median nerve at the wrist as the primary way to "prove" dysfunction of the carpal tunnel, which is located at the palm.

Provocative testing is when doctors brusquely bend their patients' wrists up and down into harsh angles and vigorously press, prod, and tap their patients' median nerves at their wrists. If a patient has the misfortune to experience pain or numbness from the doctor's actions, the doctor concludes there is a problem in the carpal tunnel (again, which is located at the palm) and that surgery will likely be required.

Think about it. Doctors do not perform this bending, pressing, tapping, and prodding at the actual site of the "tunnel" (on the palm). They "provoke" the median nerve at the wrist before it enters the carpal tunnel. They do not know if there is a problem with the carpal tunnel, or, and this is of extreme importance, the precise nature of any problem that may exist. For them, it is all speculation.

Restricting one's attention exclusively to a tiny bit of tissue that lies beyond the wrist does not make medical sense. Doctors do not carefully examine the soft tissues of their patients or listen to their complaints of pain that conflict with their preconceived notions. They are therefore unaware of what causes their patients' pain.

Electrophysiological testing is no better. Many individuals who display abnormal electrical findings do not have symptoms, and many others who do have symptoms have perfectly normal electrical findings.

What this means is that doctors have not demonstrated the need for surgery when their patients are rushed to operating rooms to have scalpels slice into their carpal tunnels. Surgery performed without diagnostic justification is surgical mutilation, a form of malpractice.

If It's Not Carpal Tunnel Syndrome, What Is It?

Restricting one's attention exclusively to a tiny bit of tissue that lies beyond the wrist does not make medical sense. As mentioned throughout this book, doctors do not carefully examine the soft tissues of their patients or listen to their complaints of pain that conflict with their preconceived notions. They are therefore unaware of what causes their patients' pain.

With very few exceptions, such as rare bony abnormalities, fractures, or temporary hormonal changes that occur during pregnancy, extensive soft tissue dysfunction is the cause of the pain. The use of lotion as a discovering or connecting agent is of vital importance to carefully examine the body tissues of the pain sufferer. When this is done, tissue dysfunction will be found throughout the entire upper extremity, from the shoulder down the arm to the elbow, wrist, and hand. The tissues of the neck, back, and chest are also very likely to be dysfunctional. Tissue dysfunction may indeed occur at the carpal tunnel, but this is merely one small part of an extensive problem. The misleading term of Carpal Tunnel Syndrome (CTS) should be replaced with the more accurate and honest one of Extensive Soft Tissue Dysfunction (ESTD).

How Does ESTD Develop?

We are told that repetitive wrist movement when we use our computer keyboard is the cause of our problems. That is why doctors prescribe wrist splints—to prevent our wrists from moving. However, if you look down when you are working at your keyboard, you will see that your wrists are not moving. It is your fingers that move repetitively.

Your fingers move repetitively because the muscles connected to them are constantly contracting. These muscles are forced to contract rapidly; 150 times a minute is a conservative estimate. I calculate that at this rate these muscles contract 9,000 times in one hour and 72,000 times in an eight-hour workday. This means that in a five-day week they contract 360,000 times, and in one month, the muscles contract 7,200,000 times.

It so happens that these overworked muscles are attached at the elbow. This is where the soft tissue dysfunction starts: at the elbow.

As these overworked muscles become increasingly unhealthy, they trigger other muscle groups to become unhealthy. Other tissue systems such as fascia and ligaments are also triggered to become unhealthy. Even the skin throughout the affected area is stimulated to become unhealthy. The problem in terms of tissue systems and areas of the body involved is truly an extensive one.

Nor does this happen overnight. It takes place gradually over a period of weeks, months, and years. It develops so gradually that our bodies are able to accommodate to the significant changes that take place. We are aware of aches and pains and stiffness here and there. At times we may complain of a stiff neck or a sore shoulder or a painful forearm, but a visit to the doctor for painkillers takes the edge off the pain, thus enabling our pain sensing center to further adjust to the continuing tissue changes.

One of the many tissues that have been stimulated to become unhealthy is the carpal ligament, the roof of the carpal tunnel. It thickens and contracts and draws the carpal bones closer together, narrowing the cross section of the carpal tunnel, thereby increasing the pressure on the median nerve.

As time goes on and it becomes increasingly thick, it presses down directly on the nerve, which lies immediately below, stressing it more and more. The ligament, and the fascia and skin overlying it, eventually becomes a thickened, hardened, adherent mass that causes even greater stress on the median nerve. As the median nerve becomes progressively stressed, pain becomes more severe.

Because doctors do not know how to properly examine their patients, they do not understand this. They fancy that tendons passing deep in the tunnel somehow swell and press the median nerve up into what they regard as a healthy carpal ligament. In order to relieve the pressure, they sever the ligament.

Bizarre, isn't it? The "gold standard" of medical care the doctors offer patients suffering from what they call carpal tunnel syndrome is to mutilate perceived healthy tissue. Some local relief of pain and other symptoms may result from surgically relieving pressure on the median nerve. However, surgical intrusion may cause nerve damage and bowing of flexor tendons, and postsurgical scarring always worsens a soft tissue problem.

Patients with the best of results are very likely to find that their fingers, hands, and arms do not have the strength or agility to return to their original occupation. Indeed, there are those, doctors tell us, whose damage from repetitive motion disorder is so severe that they are permanently disabled and will have to live the rest of their lives in pain, unable to use their hands for any gainful employment. These poor results and gloomy prognoses spring from a lack of knowledge of soft tissue dysfunction. Ignorance has led to improper treatment.

The proper treatment for this extensive problem is to normalize all the dysfunctioning tissue wherever it occurs: neck, back, shoulder, arm, forearm, hand, fingers, thumb. When this is done, the individual becomes pain-free and healthy again and can return to full-time occupation. If the occupation happens to be particularly stressful, repeat treatments can be given from time to time so the individual can remain healthy and pain-free, can continue to feel great, and can continue to perform his or her job of choice.

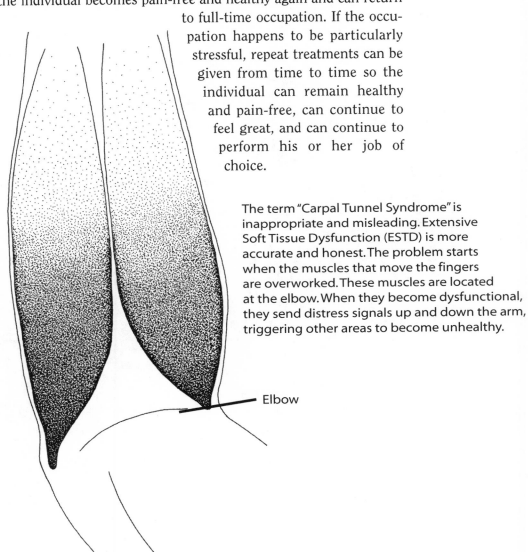

The term "Carpal Tunnel Syndrome" is inappropriate and misleading. Extensive Soft Tissue Dysfunction (ESTD) is more accurate and honest. The problem starts when the muscles that move the fingers are overworked. These muscles are located at the elbow. When they become dysfunctional, they send distress signals up and down the arm, triggering other areas to become unhealthy.

Elbow

Stressed tissues at the elbow become tight, contracted, and fibrotic.

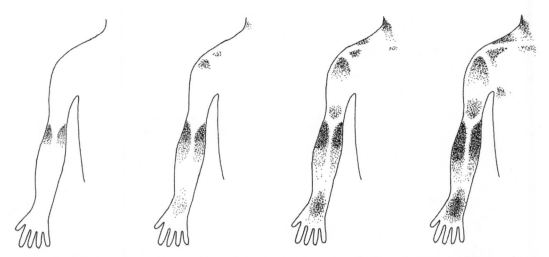

The problem that started at the elbow triggers progressive dysfunction up and down the arm.

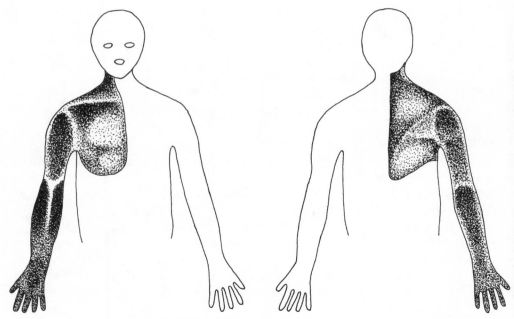

This drawing depicts fully developed ESTD. The problem that started at the elbow now extends up to the neck, back, and chest, and down to the hand. The tissues of the carpal tunnel may be affected, but they are one small area of an extensive problem. All areas must be treated if the individual is to become pain-free and healthy again. Surgery for this soft tissue problem, or *any* soft tissue problem, is inappropriate. It introduces scarring and may damage nerves and vessels. Surgery does not soften tight, contracted tissues.

The skin of an unhealthy hand is thick and tight; the creases are deep.

Under the creases lie areas of tight, contracted tissues that have to be softened so health can return.

The famous carpal tunnel

Components of the carpal tunnel

Carpal ligament
(roof of tunnel)

Carpal bones
(sides and bottom)

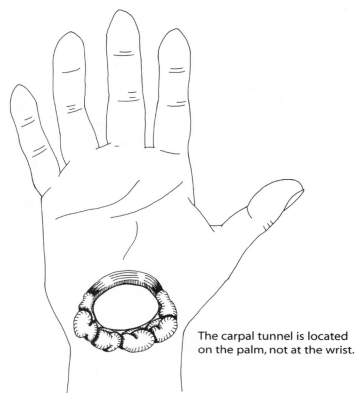

The carpal tunnel is located on the palm, not at the wrist.

Cross sections of the carpal tunnel

The important median nerve passes through the tunnel immediately below the carpal ligament. For clarity, the tendons that lie deep in the tunnel have been omitted.

Perspective view of the median nerve passing directly under the carpal ligament

Cross section of the carpal tunnel showing median nerve and the tendons that move the fingers. The median nerve passes directly under the carpal ligament. Finger tendons lie deep in the tunnel.

Perspective view of the median nerve and finger tendons as they pass directly under the carpal ligament

When stimulated by unhealthy forearm tissues, the carpal ligament thickens and contracts.

It presses down on the median nerve, squeezing and stressing it.

The contracting carpal ligament pulls on the carpal bones, narrowing the cross section of the tunnel. This increases the pressure and stress on the median nerve.

While all of this is happening, the tendons stay in place deep in the tunnel. The median nerve has been stressed by the thickened and contracted carpal ligament (that was triggered by forearm tissues), not by the deep tendons.

With effective (nonsurgical) treatment, the carpal ligament and all dysfunctioning tissues of the hand, arm, neck, back, and chest become soft, supple, and healthy again.

Soft Tissue Manipulation Treatments

Let us say that someone comes for treatment bearing the diagnosis of carpal tunnel syndrome. This is how I treat it. First of all, I set aside a block of at least two hours of uninterrupted treatment time. I frequently start my investigation of the patient's tissues at the shoulder. Lotion is applied, and I feel for tight, contracted tissue. I work down the arm, continually feeling for dysfunctioning tissue, applying additional lotion as needed. I work gently. One can work gently but still move tissues deep in the body. When tight tissues are found, they are coaxed to relax, to let go.

A process of the patient getting acquainted with his or her body begins. The gentle work awakens pain that has lain dormant for perhaps years. A variety of techniques—all gentle, all involving coaxing—is used. As the awakened pain subsides, healing has begun.

Treatment continues down the arm. The patient is usually surprised at the large amount of pain that has been stored up at the elbow. I work very gently there. The forearm reveals severely thickened and painful tissue. I work thoroughly there. Before I get to the wrist, patients frequently tell me that the pain and tingling in their hand and fingers has subsided significantly, or has gone away entirely. This surprises them greatly.

We are now at the hand. The hand is the end point, the downstream terminus of all the complex of dysfunction that lies above it. The skin of a dysfunctioning hand is thickened and tight. The joints of the palm, fingers, and thumb are bound down by thick tissue that has a hard scarlike consistency. The creases of the joints are deep, thick, and painful to light touch. The tissue just beyond the wrist, at the base of the palm, is severely thickened and feels like a piece of rigid plastic. The skin is adherent to this hard, thick area. When gently pressed, the patient frequently feels increased pain and tingling of the thumb and first two fingers.

This is the area of the carpal tunnel. Instead of cutting into it with a sharp knife as a doctor would do, in Tissue Sculpting it is gently kneaded and coaxed to relax, to soften, to become healthy again. We move on to the palm proper, and the thumb and fingers.

It is surprising how frequently, even at the very first treatment, that the patient feels a significant response to this gentle work. I have had patients tell me their pain has gone down seventy-five percent by the end of their first treatment. Some no longer have any pain and their entire arm feels lighter and more alive. Not only that, their fingers are less stiff and move in a more normal manner.

The moments have flown by. Both the patient and I are astonished that two hours have passed in a twinkling. We have made a good start. At the next visit, we will do more. We will treat the same areas, but, as they have already begun to soften and normalize, we won't have to spend as much time on them, so we can move on to the neck and back and perhaps the other arm. Wherever we find tight, contracted tissue, there is where we will treat.

Frequency of treatment depends on the severity of the problem and the patient's response to treatment. I might suggest two to three treatments the first week, reducing as soon as possible to once a week, then perhaps once every two weeks, and so on. I might want to do a recheck in three or four months to make sure there has been no return of tightness. When the patient is finally discharged, all treated areas are soft, supple, pain-free and healthy. The (former) patient now feels great! It is surprising how wonderful a person feels when his body has been properly treated.

Case History 1

Nine years ago, my wife told me that her hairstylist, Theresa, had developed severely painful arms and hands and was no longer able to work. Theresa had an appointment with the hand clinic of a particular teaching hospital the following Thursday. Theresa, I was told, was distraught by all the pain she was having and was fearful and apprehensive about her future. My wife told Theresa that I treated people with severe pain and was apparently successful because so many people called to thank me for helping them. She suggested that Theresa call me, as I might have some suggestions for her.

When I talked with her, she sobbed continuously and there was panic in her voice. She told me that her problem had developed over a two-year period and particularly involved her dominant left arm and hand. The pain had gotten so bad that she could barely lift her arm and could no longer hold a pair of scissors or a blow dryer. In addition, the constant pain was affecting her emotionally. She asked if I could tell her anything that might be of help.

I told Theresa exactly what would happen when she went to the hand clinic. The doctors would put her through all kinds of tests and examinations. Some would be uncomfortable; some would likely be excruciatingly painful. The tests and examinations would probably drag on for two or three weeks and in the end the doctors would not be able to offer her anything that would help her become healthy and pain-free again.

I told Theresa that there was a chance I might be able to help and enable her to avoid the painful and ultimately unproductive tests she would be put through at the hand clinic. I suggested that I treat her on the following Monday, Tuesday, and Wednesday. We would have three days to see if my treatments would be of significant help. If they were, then she would not have to go through the painful procedures at the hand clinic. If my treatments were not successful, then at least my findings might provide information that would help the doctors.

I would need a doctor's prescription that allowed me to examine and treat her. I suggested that she call the doctors at the hand clinic, tell them about our conversation, and ask them if they could give her a check-over the following day in order to provide me with a prescription to treat. It was my feeling that the doctors at the hand clinic would not give Theresa the prescription. It was my experience and observation that doctors did not want to lose control of a patient or a prospective patient, but maybe I would be proven wrong. My schedule was full for the following week, but I knew my patients would be pleased that someone else would have a chance to become pain-free and would not mind being rescheduled.

Theresa said that what I told her made sense and that she would call the doctors. Her voice sounded relieved. We made arrangements to meet at my office on Monday morning at nine.

I arrived at my office early on Monday to set things up. At 8:45 A.M., the phone rang. It was Theresa. She had called the doctors at the hand clinic, and they told her that it is was of extreme importance that she keep her appointment with them on Thursday, as only they had the knowledge and expertise to evaluate her problem and that under no circumstance should she do anything before they told her that she could do it. Theresa apologized for the trouble she had caused with the rescheduling of my patients. She thanked me for my time and trouble. I wished her luck, and we hung up. I felt miffed, largely because I thought I could have helped her and saved her a lot of grief.

Two weeks later, the phone rang. It was Theresa. She sounded even more distraught than before. In between her sobs, she told me that things had gone along exactly as I told her they would. The tests and exams made her pain completely unbearable. Especially horrible were the sharp needles they inserted into her already painful forearms. She told me the doctors had done all the testing but she would have to wait a week for the final consultation, when the chief doctor would tell her about their findings and conclusions and the treatments they would suggest.

Her arm and hand had become so unbearably painful that she couldn't wait the week until the final consultation. She asked if I might be able to schedule her in for anything that might reduce her pain. I reminded Theresa that I needed a prescription that would allow me to treat her. She felt confident that the doctors at the hand clinic would understand that she was hurting so badly and would gladly give her a prescription for something that might help her pain.

The next morning, I arrived at my office well before the 9:00 A.M. time we had arranged. At 8:45 the phone rang. This time it was Theresa's husband. He told me that Theresa had called the hand clinic, but they told her absolutely not to see anybody or do anything until the final consultation the following week, no matter how "uncomfortable" she was. Theresa's husband apologized. He said he knew this was the second time she had canceled. As a matter of fact, she was too embarrassed to call herself. I told Theresa's husband not to worry. I was deeply sorry she was having so much pain and wished them both luck.

A week later, the phone rang, and it was Theresa again. She said, "Bernard, you won't believe what happened at the final consultation yesterday!" She had asked her husband to accompany her to the final consultation, as she was too nervous and upset to go alone. When they were ushered into the chief doctor's office, he was seated behind his desk, attired in his white jacket, thumbing through her examination and test folder. There was a moment of silence as he finished his perusal of her reports. He then said that he was sorry and saddened to report to them that her case of carpal tunnel syndrome was so severe, that the condition of her hands and fingers was so terrible, that even surgery would not be able to help her. Her case was beyond help.

He *could* tell her that she would have to change careers. She would have to find some line of work in which she wouldn't have to use her hands. He was sorry, but there was nothing that could be done for her. Theresa then asked if the physical therapist for whom she had been requesting prescriptions might be able to help her.

"Well, yes," replied the doctor, "you might try him."

At this point, her husband got up and approached the doctor. Theresa said that her husband is a mild person but he was so angry she thought he was going to punch the doctor. "You mean to tell us that after all this time, there is nothing you can do? But that maybe the person you had us cancel twice, and probably won't even want to speak to us, might be of some help?" The doctor hurriedly (at last) wrote out the prescription, and they left. Her husband did not strike the doctor.

When Theresa came for her first treatment, her face was drawn with pain. She moved her arms and hands guardedly and held the fingers of her hands open and outstretched. She talked slowly and seemed on the verge of tears. She told me her experience at the hand clinic had been a terrible one and that she was deeply depressed and worried about what they had told her. She had been a hairstylist for nineteen years and it was a career she loved. It was the only thing she knew how to do or wanted to do.

After the final consultation at the hand clinic, she and her husband had discussed alternative careers in which she wouldn't have to use her hands. The only thing they could think of was some sort of day care for children. But even with something like that she would have to pick up a child, which presently she was unable to do.

I found that the tissues of her upper and mid-back, her neck, both shoulders, arms, forearms, wrists, hands, and fingers, in addition to the tissues of her left anterior torso, were spasmed, contracted, thickened, fibrotic, and extremely painful to even very mild palpation. The tissues of her left upper extremity were more severely affected than her right. The skin overlying these areas was thickened, adherent, and very painful to light touch. She couldn't bend the fingers of her left hand, or hold anything in them. It caused her great pain to drive her car, as she couldn't grip the steering wheel in a normal fashion with either hand.

I worked on Theresa for three hours. At the end of this time, she said she felt "great." She was able to bend the fingers of both hands and reported that the pain in her arms and hands was down seventy-five percent. She was extremely pleased with the results of the first visit.

When she came by the next day for her second treatment, she reported that she had been able to drive home after yesterday's treatment with her hands and fingers gripping the steering wheel of her car in a completely normal fashion, without pain.

It is sad that the medical community has so little understanding of the underlying cause of body dysfunction such that the neurologists, orthopedic surgeons, and rehabilitation specialists of a prestigious medical teaching hospital doomed Theresa to a life of progressive, crippling pain. Instead, when she received appropriate care, she rapidly became healthy, happy, and pain-free again.

I worked on Theresa daily the first week in three-hour sessions. During that week, there was some flare-up of pain here and there, but by the end of the week she was feeling no pain, except an occasional twinge.

Although Theresa was feeling well by that time, she was worried about her return to work the following week. She had not been able to work at all for several days. Her workdays for the previous two or three months had been nightmarish with pain. However, when she came by for treatment following her first day of return to work, she reported that she had been able to perform her regular duties all day without pain, except for a little twinge in her left palm.

I continued to work on Theresa for the next four months at rapidly decreasing treatment frequency. There were times when she had minor flare-ups of pain, but for the most part, the treatments were directed toward reducing areas of remaining contracted tissue so they would not retrigger pain in the future.

When we discontinued treatment at the end of the four months, Theresa was completely pain-free and feeling very well. Her tissues were soft, supple, and she no longer felt emotionally stressed. She had begun to lift weights again, and she was able to continue her career as a hairstylist.

It is sad that the medical community has so little understanding of the underlying cause of body dysfunction such that the neurologists, orthopedic surgeons, and rehabilitation specialists of a prestigious medical teaching hospital doomed Theresa to a life of progressive, crippling pain. Instead, when she received appropriate care, she rapidly became healthy, happy, and pain-free again.

I sent regular reports about Theresa's recovery to the doctor— to the one who had told her there was nothing that could be done, that she would have to change careers, and would have to live the rest of her life in pain. However, he did not have even the professional curiosity to ask me to show him what I had done to help her so he could use the information to help his other patients.

Although it has been nine years since I treated Theresa, she continues to do extremely well, to be pain-free, and is feeling great.

Case History 2

An article in a local paper described the plight of a young woman who had severe carpal tunnel syndrome of both wrists. Her condition was so painful and critical that surgery was scheduled for both wrists in two weeks. She had no medical insurance and was in the process of selling her small business to pay for the surgery.

I phoned her and asked if she would be interested in trying non-surgical treatment for her carpal tunnel problem. I told her there would be no charge, but I would need a doctor's prescription allowing me to treat her. She said she was very interested and that there would be no problem in getting the doctor's prescription. She had a wonderful doctor who would be willing to try anything that might help her.

She arrived at the appointed time bearing the prescription. She informed me that her doctor wanted to speak with me before I started any treatment. I immediately called him. He told me that under no circumstance was I to do anything that would interfere with the surgery that was scheduled for his patient. I assured him that I understood what he was saying. He said that I could then go ahead and treat her.

The first thing I noticed was her wrist splints. They were filthy. She had been wearing them for several months (if worn continuously for more than a week or two, splints cause immobilization problems). She had been told to wear one on each wrist at all times. I learned that her fingers, hands, and forearms caused her continual and severe pain and tingling, and that any movement increased the pain to an even higher level. Her hands had grown weak, and she had difficulty doing the simplest task. Driving was dangerous because the pain, weakness, and the cumbersome splints made gripping the steering wheel difficult.

I removed the splints and noted that her fingers, hands, wrists, and forearms were swollen and painful to the lightest touch. The joints of her fingers and palms were thickened, and it was difficult and painful for her to move them even slightly. Her right hand was more painful than her left.

I treated her three times the first week in three-hour sessions. At the end of the first session, she stated that there was less pain and tingling in both hands and wrists, and she could move her fingers more easily.

When she came in for her second session, she was not wearing her wrist splints. Her hands and arms were so comfortable that she felt she didn't need them, she said. She reported that she was able to grip the steering wheel of her car in a "near-normal" fashion. At the end of the second session, she stated that there was no longer any pain or tingling in her left wrist and hand, and only a small amount of pain in her right forearm, and the only tingling was in her right forefinger.

When she came in for her third session, she reported that she was "feeling a lot better all around" and had even felt well enough to resume horseback riding after the previous session, and she had canceled her surgery. She stated that there was "barely noticeable" pain in her right forearm, and a "slight tingling" in the last two joints of her right forefinger. At the end of the third session, she stated that she no longer had any pain or tingling in either hand, wrist, or forearm.

We still had a lot of work to do. Considerable contracted tissue remained, and there was some grip weakness that had to be resolved. I advised her to avoid horseback riding until after discharge, as we didn't want to contend with additional problems that might result from her being thrown from a horse. We agreed to continue our three-times-a-week treatment schedule.

I sent a preliminary report to her doctor describing her improved status, and she went back to him the following week for a recheck. She could hardly wait to show him how improved she was. When she returned for treatment following her doctor's visit, I asked how things went. She told me that she had proudly demonstrated how she could move her hands and arms freely and without pain, and that she had canceled her surgery appointments. I asked what her doctor had said. Her reply: "He didn't say anything."

I continued treating her at decreasing frequency for the next six weeks. She was then discharged, pain- and symptom-free. I continued reporting to her doctor as treatments continued, but did not receive any communication from him. I thought he would be interested in finding out what I had done that allowed his patient to avoid those drastic and expensive surgeries, but apparently I was wrong.

Case History 3

A young woman stopped by my office. She had recently seen a TV program that had her worried. The program described the symptoms of carpal tunnel syndrome and warned viewers that carpal tunnel syndrome can become irreversible if treatment is delayed too long. She told me that she worked for the post office and that her job was to continuously feed envelopes into a mechanical device throughout the workday. Over the past year, her hands and arms had become increasingly painful and stiff. Recently the pain had become so severe, and her fingers had become so stiff, that she could no longer ignore the problem. The TV program had convinced her that she had carpal tunnel syndrome and that her condition was now irreversible.

She had an appointment with a doctor who specialized in carpal tunnel syndrome and was going to see him in a few days. In the meantime, someone I had helped suggested she contact me. I told her that I would need a doctor's prescription to treat her. She said she would get one the following week from the carpal tunnel syndrome specialist. We arranged for her to see me immediately following her doctor's appointment.

She arrived for her treatment in a state of panic. Her fears had been justified. She did have carpal tunnel syndrome, and it was indeed severe. I noticed that she was wearing a wrist splint on each wrist. The doctor said that, because of the severity of her problem, she was to wear the splints at all times, day and night for the next three weeks. He had written a note to her supervisor, stating that it was important for his patient to completely rest her hands and wrists for three weeks and she was not to report for work during this time. She was to return to him at the end of the three-week period for reassessment. When she asked the doctor for a prescription allowing me to treat her, he at first refused, but when she insisted he finally signed one.

She was alarmed, because the doctor said she had waited so long that her carpal tunnel syndrome was now severe. She was concerned about her job because it was a busy season and her supervisor would not be pleased about her absence of three weeks. She dreaded the idea of wearing the uncomfortable wrist splints for three weeks, day and night.

I removed the splints and examined her hands and arms. The tissues of both upper extremities were tight and contracted, but not so much as to incite panic. I had examined and successfully treated tissues that were considerably more dysfunctional than hers. I told her that, although no guarantee could be given, I thought there was a good chance she could achieve a complete recovery.

I worked on her fingers, hands, arms, shoulders, and back for three hours. At the end of this time, the tissues of those areas were appreciably looser and less painful. She was now hopeful that she could be successfully treated. She felt so much better that she thought she didn't need the wrist splints. She asked what I thought. I told her that if the doctor said to wear the splints for three weeks that she had better do so. I added that if it were me that had to wear the splints, I would throw them in the trash can, but she should follow the doctor's orders.

When she returned for her next treatment two days later, she told me that following our first session she had stopped by the doctor's office with the splints he had sold her (she had to pay cash for them) and asked for her money back. There was some reluctance to take back the splints and to return her money, but she had insisted, saying that "because of the good work of Mr. Schatz" she no longer needed them. Finally, her money was returned and the splints were taken back. She continued to do her post office duties and was fairly comfortable even after eight hours of work, and, although she experienced some pain in her hands and arms, "It was nothing like before."

We continued sessions three days a week for the next three weeks. We then reduced their frequency to two days a week for the following three weeks, then down to once a week for a month. Her fingers, hands, and forearms responded well, and rapidly became pain-free. Much of the treatment emphasis was directed toward her upper arms (particularly her right) and her neck. During the entire treatment period, she continued to work full shifts with the mechanical device she had to deal with. At the end of this time, she was discharged from treatment, pain- and symptom-free, and feeling great.

She called two months later. She was experiencing some tightness in her shoulders and arms, accompanied by a little pain, and wanted me to work on them before things got worse. I noted some return of tissue tightness and contraction. These responded rapidly and in three two-hour sessions she was once again discharged from treatment.

Another call came six months later. She had worked continuously without pain or discomfort until a few days earlier. The workload with the mechanical device she had to contend with had gotten particularly heavy and there was some return of tightness and some pain in her arms and forearms. Her fingers and hands had continued to do well. A few more treatments and she was pain-free and supple again.

I reported her progress to the doctor—the one that specialized in carpal tunnel syndrome—who had signed the prescription allowing me to treat. I also called him several times, trying to arrange an appointment so I could discuss with him my treatment methods that had nonsurgically reversed and normalized the tissues of someone he had diagnosed as having severe carpal tunnel syndrome. But he never had time to talk with me. Nor did he ever refer a patient for treatment of carpal tunnel syndrome, despite the significant recovery this patient had made *without* wearing uncomfortable wrist splints or without being subjected to other medical treatments, including surgery, that usually follow the diagnosis of severe carpal tunnel syndrome.

Case History 4

A sixty-two-year-old woman came to me for treatment of her painful hands. A friend had told her of my work, and she had a prescription allowing me to treat.

When I took her case history, I learned that carpal tunnel surgery had been performed on both her hands, one surgery on her left hand, and two on her right. Unfortunately, the surgeries had not alleviated the pain of either hand. Her right hand had been more painful, which was why the surgeons had tried a second surgery two years prior to her appointment with me.

She told me that in addition to the pain, both her hands had grown increasingly weak. She had difficulty manipulating keys, holding glassware, or using a pen or pencil. Following each surgery, she received physical therapy consisting of warm paraffin dips, stretches, and exercises, but those procedures had not helped her pain or weakness.

She was surprised when I applied lotion to her right shoulder and began palpating the tissues there, because none of the doctors or therapists had touched those tissues. She was further surprised at all the tightness and pain there. I let her feel the lotioned skin of her shoulder, arm, and forearm so she could see how thick the tissues were in those areas and how painful they were to her light touch. We found contracted tissues in her hand. The skin was thick and drawn tightly across the palm. The surgical scarring on her palm was adherent to the tissues under it, and her fingers were stiff. I found similar tissue dysfunction on her left side, but not to the same extent.

I treated her daily for two weeks. The first week, I concentrated on her right upper extremity, and the second week on her left side. She responded rapidly to treatment, and at the end of the two-week period she no longer had any pain in either hand, her strength had improved significantly, and she was able to use both hands in a normal manner.

She was delighted with the results and felt she did not need further treatment, although I still felt tight tissues. I told her to call me if any symptoms recurred. No call ever came. I sent a report to the doctor who signed her prescription, describing her dramatic response to my treatments. No call came from him, either.

Why the Silence from the Doctors?

I was invited to speak to an organization of nurses about my approach to the treatment of carpal tunnel syndrome. I had helped the sister of one of their members, which was how they knew of my work. At the meeting, I discussed what I found to be the cause of carpal tunnel syndrome and my approach to treating it. I told them I was surprised I had never received another referral from a doctor to whom I had returned a patient successfully treated for previously untreatable symptoms. Not one doctor had bothered to ask me what I had done to help a patient previously judged to be "unhelpable."

I asked the nurses, all of whom worked closely with doctors, why the doctors never made more referrals? They were unanimous in their response:

- The doctors did not want to lose control of their patients.

- The doctors did not want to admit that they had previously been wrong in their treatment approach.

- The doctors did not want to allow someone outside their profession to come up with something better.

- The doctors were running a business and didn't want to lose revenue.

- The doctors had forgotten why they had become doctors, which was to help people first and foremost.

Soft Tissue Manipulation Techniques

I do not know if you have been having problems for an extended time or if your symptoms have surfaced recently. Perhaps you have been subjected to one or more surgeries. Each case has to be treated on an individual basis, so only a generalized approach can be described here.

For purposes of illustration, I am going to assume your problem is primarily with the tissues of your right upper extremity. The tissues of your neck, upper back, and chest, as well as your left upper extremity, are probably also involved. Refer to "Migraine and Muscle Contraction Headaches" and "Frozen Shoulder" for soft tissue manipulation suggestions for those areas.

Keep in mind that as your fingers explore and investigate your tissues, they are at the same time treating those tissues. The more your fingers investigate, the more they treat.

We will concentrate here on your shoulder down to your fingertips. Before you start treatment, try this: wiggle the fingers of your affected hand. Wiggle them as fast as you can. It is likely they move slowly, stiffly, and painfully. Now wiggle the fingers of your "better" hand. It is likely these fingers move more freely and wiggle faster than your affected hand. We will recheck these movements following your treatment.

Get into a comfortable sitting position with a towel-covered pillow on your lap and a container of lotion and a cup of warm water next to you. Warm the lotion, if you wish.

Place your forearm and hand on the pillow. This will help to relax the tissues of your upper extremity, making your treatment more effective. Don't hold your elbow away from your body, as this will tense your tissues. Instead, let your arm go slack against your body; this will greatly assist you in your examination and treatment. Keep in mind that as your fingers explore and investigate your tissues, they are at the same time treating those tissues. The more your fingers investigate, the more they treat.

With your left hand, apply a liberal amount of lotion to your shoulder. Use finger and thumb sweeps over your entire shoulder muscle (the deltoid), then doubled-finger circles, and nudges. Let your fingers get acquainted with the tissues there. Are they hard and stringy? Do you find pain there? Adjust the amount of lotion by wiping with a towel, so your sweeps, circles, and nudges have more grip, enabling you to sense the underlying tissues a bit differently. You want to get as much information about those tissues as possible. Explore the muscle, top to bottom, side to side.

Pincer the deltoid up at its very top between your thumb and forefinger. Rock it with push-pulls. Go down its entirety to where it attaches, about halfway down your arm, then back up and proceed downward with thumb kneadings. Continue with this up-to-down pattern. Follow the bands of tissues that you feel inside, that run down the length of the muscle. Keep looking for tight and painful areas. This is your first session; you will be busy with all sorts of discoveries as you proceed.

Turn your attention to the skin overlying your deltoid. Explore with skin ripples. Can you find thickened areas of skin? Painful areas? Now try skin graspings. Do you find areas adherent to underlying tissues? Any painful areas? Carefully check the area where the deltoid attaches; you are apt to find thickened, dysfunctioning skin there.

Finish investigation and treatment of your deltoid tissues with overall kneadings. I wager your deltoid is now considerably looser and more supple.

Move down to your biceps tissues. Let's start with the skin. Apply lotion. Grasp the muscle with your fingers on the outside, and your thumb on the inside, up into your armpit. Sweep with thumb to the fingers. Look for thick, crinkly skin; these are signs of skin dysfunction. Remember, wherever you find areas of skin dysfunction, you will invariably find tissue problems underneath that need treatment, so always examine the skin carefully. Do you find painful areas, or areas that become painful after gentle exploration? Use skin graspings, circles, and floats.

When you have examined your skin to your satisfaction, turn your attention to the deeper tissues. Thumb side-to-sides will be useful on the inside tissues that run down from your armpit to the lower attachment of the muscle just beyond the elbow. Use your fingers for back-and-forths on the outside tissues. It is likely that you will find hard, painful, wirelike bands that need softening and normalizing, particularly toward the lower attachment of the muscle. Use single- and multiple-finger circles. Follow with thumb circles.

Pincer the muscle and perform push-pulls. Finish with a good over-all kneading.

You are ready to turn your attention to the tissues on the opposite side of the biceps; these are the tissues associated with the triceps muscle (the biceps bends your elbow; the triceps straightens it). Start again with skin exploration using skin ripples and graspings. It is likely you will find considerable crinkly skin overlying the triceps. Explore the deeper tissues with nudges, waves, and circles.

It is possible that in your treatment so far, you found areas that triggered sensations down into your hand and fingers, such as increased pain, tingling, or numbness. As you proceed, these hand and finger sensations will undoubtedly increase dramatically because you are now ready to explore and treat the tissues that are primarily responsible for the problems doctors misleadingly call carpal tunnel syndrome.

You are now going to work on your forearm. The forearm muscles and associated tissues are attached close to the elbow. They move your thumb and fingers, and are the tissues that get over-worked. Be prepared to find considerable amounts of overt and hidden pain in these tissues.

Apply some lotion to the muscle bulge that lies on the thumb side of your forearm. These muscles straighten your fingers and thumb. Work the skin overlying these tissues; thumb sweeps are good. Treat the skin thoroughly, from above the elbow, down to the wrist. Then turn your attention to the tissues underneath. Start with pincering the muscle bulge and gently rock with push-pulls. Follow the bulge from where it starts above the elbow down to where it separates into the various thumb and finger tendons. Then try thumb and finger circles, back-and-forths, and nudges. Learn to trust your fingers; let them suggest what patterns you should use. Look for painful, contracted muscle bands that lead downward. Track these with back-and-forths.

You will likely find a particularly hard, painful band that starts just above the bump at your elbow joint and passes down into your hand next to the bump at your wrist joint.

Most likely, you will find extensive tight, contracted, and extremely painful tissues on this side of your forearm. Are you surprised at what you have found so far? And you haven't even gotten to your hand yet!

You are now ready to explore and treat the other forearm bulge. This contains the muscles that bend your thumb and fingers. Additional surprises await you here. Apply lotion, and be particularly gentle, because these tissues are likely to be more tender than those of the finger straighteners. When you explore these tissues, are you aware of sensations that shoot up your arm, and down into your hand? By the way, how is your hand feeling? Chances are your hand and fingers are feeling better with less pain and numbness. Does this surprise you?

Your first treatment is a "get-acquainted" session. When you have gotten acquainted with the tissues of your forearm, you are ready to move down to your hand, fingers, and thumb.

The first thing is to simply look at your hand and fingers. Look at the skin of your palm. Is it drawn tight? Are the creases thick and deep? Does the skin have a callused appearance, as if you have done a lot of yard work? These are all indications of tissue dysfunction— of an unhealthy hand. How about the fingers; do they look swollen? Are the creases at their joints thickened and deep? What about the color of your hand and fingers? Does the skin have a dark cast to it? Do the joints of your fingers have a shiny grapelike appearance? These are more indications of dysfunction.

When you straighten your thumb and fingers as far as they will go, can you feel the skin overlying your palm stretched tightly? Run your examining fingers over the surface of your hand. Does the skin feel rough? Examine the area of your palm that lies just beyond your wrist, between the bulges of your thumb and pinky finger. Nudge this tissue with your forefinger. Does it resist? It is likely that you will find the skin here to be thick and adherent to underlying tissues. Press down on it with your examining forefinger. Does this maneuver cause increased pain and numbness in your thumb and fingers?

This is the area of the carpal tunnel. A surgeon would cut and mutilate that tissue and charge you thousands of dollars for the disservice. You will soon find, however, that the thickened tissue can be softened and normalized, can become healthy again, by gentle, humane treatment.

Let's treat that tissue. You will be able to identify it easily because it will be thick and hard with a plastic-like feel, and will have an oval shape. Apply some lotion to it. Begin the softening process with gentle nudges applied at its border. Go completely around its border with nudges that are directed toward its center. Now try thumb sweeps over the tissue. Experiment with varying amounts of lotion to get just the effect you want. Take your time.

If a surgeon has already mutilated the tissue, the problem has become more complicated, but the outcome for success is still good. It will take more work, however, because you will have to soften tissue that has been surgically scarred.

Use your forefinger for circles and back-and-forths. As you work on this tissue, you are likely to experience increased pain and numbness in your thumb and fingers. These sensations are temporary. Bring the tips of your thumb and pinky finger together; this will put some slack on the carpal tunnel tissues, enabling you to knead them. Pincer and apply back-and-forths and circles. Wipe off all the lotion and repeat the previously applied techniques; this will provide you with more variations and greater effect.

By this time, these tissues should have begun to soften, and you can finish the treatment here with skin ripplings. Are you pleased with the results of your treatment so far? I hope so. Do your thumb and fingers feel better?

The treatment of your hand can proceed in different directions: you can move out to the bulge of either your thumb or pinky finger. Or you might extend your palm treatment to your fingers. Once again, there is no cookbook formula.

Let's select the thumb. Work up the large bulge of your thumb. Use thumb probes, circles, and back-and-forths as you look for tight, hard bands that run from the joint of the bulge (at the wrist) into the thumb proper. Pincer the web of the thumb with back-and-forths and circles. Look for hard bands in there; these may be severely painful. Now go back and examine the joint at the base of the thumb bulge; this is the first thumb joint. Pincer it with your examining thumb on the palm side, and the examining forefinger opposite it (on the top-side of your hand). Perform push-and-pulls. You may find excruciatingly painful areas in the joint; if so, be sure to return to treat these

Joints of the thumb

Third joint

Second joint

First joint

some time in the future. It is important to resolve joint dysfunction there.

Now treat the second and third thumb joints. Work the joints with the tip of your examining thumb, performing circles and back-and-forths. Look for hard, fibrotic tissue that lies deep in the joint creases.

Go back to the smaller pinky finger bulge. It is likely you will find considerably less dysfunctioning tissue than you did in the thumb bulge. Explore and treat as you did with the thumb bulge.

Now treat the skin overlying your entire palm. It will be difficult to ripple the skin because of the nature of the terrain and because the skin is likely to be tightly adherent to the tissues beneath it. Try some thumb sweeps with varying amounts of lotion. Then wipe off all the lotion and perform small circles over all the skin creases; this will help to loosen the skin and free it from its adherent bonds. Then go back to thumb sweeps on the unlotioned skin. Perform the sweeps in all directions. I think you will find that your skin is now noticeably looser. Are you surprised that improvement can come so quickly?

Turn your attention to the deeper tissues of your palm, including the joints there. Pincer all joints with the tip of your examining thumb on the palm and your examining forefinger opposite, on the top of your hand. Loosen the joints with push-and-pulls, thumb probes, and circles. Alternate these maneuvers until you feel the palm joints loosening. You have likely found thick, painful tissues that prevent your palm joints from moving freely. You will be pleasantly surprised to find how quickly these tissues soften, and your hand becomes supple and healthy again.

You are almost finished with the treatment of your hand. Treat the joints of your fingers with pincering back-and-forths and circles. Perform short thumb sweeps along all the joint creases. Try to ripple the skin overlying these creases. This will help to soften and release the skin from underlying joint structures.

Now go to the top side of your hand. Ripple the skin there. Push-pull the joints of your hand with your thumb now topside. You may find some severely painful joint tissue that will need further treatment.

Finish the treatment of your upper extremity by going back up to your shoulder and jiggle and gently slap all the tissues from your shoulder on down to your fingertips. Enjoy the feeling of looseness and suppleness that one treatment has brought to your tissues.

Do you remember how you wiggled your fingers just before you started the treatment of your arm and hand? Now try it again, after treatment. Wiggle the fingers of your treated hand. Notice how much freer they are, and how quickly they move back and forth. Compare with the wiggles of your "better hand." It is likely that these cannot move as quickly; this is after just *one* treatment.

Continue with self-treatment sessions, and all your tissues will become soft, supple, healthy, and pain-free once again.

Chronic Pain

Doctors declare pain to be chronic when it has lasted three to six months. Sufferers are then told it is irreversible. They are given "pain medication" and sent to pain management centers, where pain sufferers are instructed to live with the pain they will suffer for the rest of their lives.

How sad that doctors do not understand that body and headache pain is a reflection of soft tissue dysfunction, and, since it is possible to treat and reverse tissue dysfunction, the resulting pain is also reversible. People do not have to suffer pain, certainly not for the rest of their lives.

Chronic pain occurs when the tissues of the body are allowed to become tight, contracted, and fibrotic. Pain will last as long as the tissue dysfunction remains untreated, whether this is three to six months, three to six years, or the entirety of the sufferer's life.

When properly treated, the early stages of tissue spasm do not develop into the later stages of contraction and fibrosis, so chronic pain will not occur. However, even the later stages of tissue dysfunction can be effectively treated and normalized, so the individual can become pain-free and healthy again.

Case History

A woman stopped by my office and asked if I could help her. She said she had been suffering severe chronic pain for eleven years. The pain had developed gradually and seemed to start a few months after a severe emotional trauma. The pain had become increasingly intense as the years passed. In addition to the excruciating pain, her body was growing stiffer, and she suffered from debilitating fatigue. She was concerned that, the way things were going, she would soon end up in a wheelchair.

She told me that she also suffered from severe depression. Not only that, but because of the distracting pain, she was finding it increasingly difficult to concentrate her thoughts.

For the past few years, the pain had become unbearable. There was not a single minute she did not suffer severe body pain and headaches. She described her life as a "living hell." She had been to several doctors over the years, but none had been able to help her. All told her the same thing: "Nothing more can be done. You will have to learn to live with your pain."

But she had never given up. She had tried everything and anything that might help her: chiropractic, acupuncture, massage, herbs, yoga, meditation. Some had helped a little, some not at all. But there was always hope in the back of her mind that someday she would find something that would give her real relief.

I told her there was a possibility that I might be able to help her, but I would need a doctor's prescription that would allow me to treat her. She said she would get one, and we set up an appointment.

When she came for our first session, I found that her scalp was drawn as tight as a drumhead, completely immovable, and terribly painful. As I gently palpated down her neck, I found that those tissues were intensely tender and sensitive to very light touch, as were the tissues of her entire back, abdomen, shoulders, both arms, both legs, gluteal area, and anterior trunk. Her entire body was tight, contracted, and painful.

It took me well over two hours to preliminarily check her body. Even though I was as gentle as possible, she cried out several times because of the extreme pain. I told her that, although I couldn't guarantee anything, I thought there was a chance I could help her. She said she was eager to try.

We started a healing venture that lasted a year and a half. I treated her three times a week in two- to three-hour sessions for the first four months. The sessions were then reduced to twice a week, then once a week, then once every two weeks, then once a month, then once every two months, until final discharge.

The first month of treatment was an agony for both of us. She cried out loudly throughout each treatment session because of the increased pain that was stirred up with even the lightest touch. I expected someone to knock on the door to see if everything was all right. Yet she continued to return for more treatment, because following each session her body was a little looser and the pain was a little less severe.

Two months after treatment started, she came in on a Monday and said that a miracle had happened over the weekend. She had gone one whole day without any pain. She considered this to be a miracle. She couldn't get over it. It was the first time in years that she had been without pain.

Thus, it continued over the next several months. Gradually, her body softened, the days without pain became more frequent, and the level of the pain diminished. Her depression began to clear, and she was able to focus her thoughts once again. She noticed that she was less fatigued.

There came a time when she no longer had any pain. All that remained was tissue tightness. We continued to work on the remaining tightness, until eventually that too was resolved. Her body was soft, supple, and free of pain. She was healthy again.

Prior to my treatments, she had been unable to work, but now she was able to get a full-time job. Her whole quality of life had changed.

When we had reduced to one treatment every two months, she became aware that at times of stress her body would begin to tighten. She learned to back away from the stress so her body wouldn't continue to tighten. A year and a half after starting, she was discharged from treatment. I told her to feel free to call me for any reason whatsoever. No call came.

I checked with her one year later. She was continuing to do fine. She did feel that she always had to be aware that stress had a tendency to retighten her body. But now that her body had been made soft and supple, she had a means of becoming aware of the first sign of retightening and was able to deal with it before it got worse.

If this woman had believed all the doctors who had told her that her chronic pain was irreversible, she never would have tried to find something that would end her pain and suffering. If she had believed her doctors, she would still be living her nightmare. It is unfortunate that there are so many more who do believe their doctors, and because of their misplaced trust they continue to exist in their living hell.

Soft Tissue Manipulation Techniques

When one suffers from what doctors call chronic pain, the entire body is usually affected. If you are one of these individuals, you have a challenging task ahead of you. I suggest that you start by examining and treating your upper extremities. Refer to "Carpal Tunnel Syndrome" for soft tissue manipulation techniques. When the tissues of your arms and hands have become normalized and free of pain, you will be better able to treat other areas of your body that may be affected.

Dizziness

Doctors associate dizziness with eye, ear, or brain disturbances. If problems in these areas cannot be found and dizziness continues, the patients are told that nothing more can be done.

However, that's not the view of Tissue Sculpting. Individuals who have soft tissue problems involving the upper back, neck, and scalp may complain of dizziness. The level of dizziness can range from mild to severe. I became aware of the relationship many years ago, when patients I treated for upper back and neck pain would, from time to time, also complain of bouts of dizziness. As their soft tissue problems were resolved, their symptoms of dizziness went away. One case was particularly dramatic.

Case History

Several years ago, I was working in a large rehabilitation facility. I received a call from a physical therapy supervisor in another unit. She had just learned of a young woman who was being treated by neurologists for profound dizziness. The dizziness was so severe that the patient required the assistance of two people, one on either side, to be able to take even a few steps.

The neurologists were convinced that such severe symptoms had to be caused by a brain tumor, but after extensive and repeated tests and examinations, the tumor had not been found. Further tests were planned. The supervisor had recalled that I had mentioned to her that dizziness could be caused by soft tissue dysfunction. She said that if I was interested, she could get a prescription allowing me to treat the patient.

I was interested, the prescription was granted, and treatment began that afternoon. When I examined the young woman, I found that the tissues of her upper back, neck, and scalp were extremely tight, contracted, and extremely tender to mild palpation. I learned that three months before her dizziness started, she had experienced a severe emotional trauma.

The patient responded rapidly to treatment. The symptoms of pain, tightness, and dizziness diminished as her tissues became softened and normalized. In two weeks, she was discharged from the facility, completely free of dizziness.

The patient responded rapidly to treatment. The symptoms of pain, tightness, and dizziness diminished as her tissues became softened and normalized. In two weeks, she was discharged from the facility, completely free of dizziness.

By the way, the neurologists never did bother to contact me to find out what I had done to so dramatically help their patient. I wonder what "other tests" they had in mind?

Soft Tissue Manipulation Techniques

The primary areas to be treated are the scalp, face, neck, and upper back. Review "Migraine and Muscle Contraction Headaches," and treat as indicated.

Dowager's Hump

"Dowager's hump" is a lay term describing the unsightly hump of tissue overlying the spinal column at the upper back that one sees occasionally on women of varying age. The hump is not caused by a distortion of the vertebrae, and is usually dismissed by doctors—if it is noticed at all—as being nothing more than an accumulation of fat.

However, if this tissue is properly examined, it will be found to be composed of thickened, contracted, and fibrotic tissue. The skin overlying this area is thick, painful, and adherent to underlying tissues. If the tissues above, below, and to either side of the hump are palpated, they also will be found to be contracted, fibrotic, and painful.

In other words, a dowager's hump is really an area of soft tissue dysfunction and, furthermore, it is an indication that there are other extensive areas of soft tissue dysfunction. It is important that the dysfunctioning tissue of a dowager's hump be treated and normalized along with the extensive areas that contributed to its formation.

Patients do not come to me with dowager's hump as a presenting symptom. It is more of a flag, an indicator, of global dysfunction. Therefore, a case history for dowager's hump will not be presented.

Soft Tissue Manipulation Techniques

Treatment consists of normalizing the tissues associated with it: the neck, upper and mid-back, and both upper extremities. For soft tissue manipulation techniques, refer to "Migraines and Muscle Contraction Headaches" and "Carpal Tunnel Syndrome."

Dupuytren's Contracture

Dupuytren's contracture is a progressive disorder of the hand in which a nodule forms in the palm and the fingers are gradually pulled tightly onto the palm. The individual is unable to straighten them, and it becomes increasingly difficult to use the hand in a normal manner.

Dupuytren's contracture does not respond to drugs, stretching, or exercise. Surgery is crude and results in the formation of scar tissue and possible nerve damage. The hand is unable to perform precise movements. If the individual is unfortunate enough to be a musician, a change of careers is very likely.

Case History

A woman called and said she had Dupuytren's contracture. Her doctor told her surgery would be required. She had heard of my work and wondered if I might be able to help her avoid surgery. I told her to get a prescription that would allow me to examine and treat, and we set up an appointment.

When I examined her, I found the characteristic nodule in the palm of her right hand, and noted that three of her fingers were curled tightly. She was unable to straighten them. I also noted tight, contracted tissues throughout both upper extremities.

She responded well to treatment. The nodule rapidly softened, and in six weeks all tissues were supple and healthy. When discharged from treatment, the nodule was completely gone and she could extend all fingers freely and easily.

Soft Tissue Manipulation Techniques

For appropriate soft tissue manipulation techniques, refer to "Carpal Tunnel Syndrome."

Ear Pain

Ear pain can be caused by a number of problems, infectious to neurologic. At times, even though doctors have explored and ruled out every possible source known to them, the patient continues to suffer. The pain of these individuals is likely caused by soft tissue dysfunction.

Case History

I received a call from a woman who said her seventy-three-year-old mother was suffering excruciating pain in her left ear. It was so severe and distracting that her mother could no longer use her walker to get about. The pain had continued over a three-week period. Her mother had been examined by several doctors, including an ear, nose, and throat specialist, and a neurologist, but the cause of pain had not been discovered.

The caller had heard of my work and wondered if I could help. I told her I would need a doctor's consent that would allow me to examine and treat her mother. She said she would obtain one, and we set up an appointment. Because her mother was so incapacitated by her pain, I agreed to treat her at their home.

When I arrived for the first treatment, I found the patient seated in a chair with her head tilted to the left. She was cradling her head in her

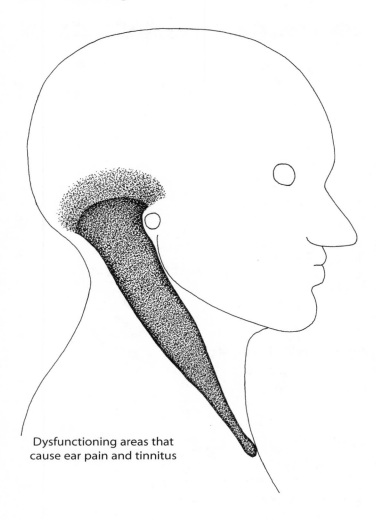

Dysfunctioning areas that
cause ear pain and tinnitus

left hand and was moaning with pain.

I found that her scalp was drawn tight and was painful to light palpation. The tissues of her face were thickened and fibrotic, as were the tissues at her upper back (i.e., the trapezius muscle). But most involved were the muscles at the front of her neck, the sternomastoids (full name: sternocleidomastoids). The left one was more affected than the right, particularly where it attached just behind her left ear. At the point of attachment, it was hard, thick, and fibrotic. Touching the area lightly caused her to cry out and to hold her head more guardedly.

I worked on the affected tissues with great care, and as I did so, the pain eased and her body relaxed. I treated her three times a week until I discharged her two weeks later. At that time, she no longer experienced any pain, and the tight and contracted tissues had softened significantly.

What was thought to be pain in her ear was really pain caused by soft tissue dysfunction close to her ear. When this was properly treated, the pain went away.

Soft Tissue Manipulation Techniques

The primary area of soft tissue dysfunction that underlies ear pain is where the sternomastoid muscle attaches just behind the ear. Other areas of soft tissue dysfunction that likely contribute to ear pain are the scalp, face, and upper back.

Lie on your back with your head comfortably supported by pillows. Arrange them so your head is tilted forward, this will produce some slack in your sternomastoids. Let us assume that your left ear is the painful one. You will turn your head to the left; this will further relax the muscle where it attaches behind your left ear.

Slip your right hand under your head so the palm of your hand supports the weight of your head. This will free your fingers and thumb to explore and treat. Start your treatment at the area of attachment with your first and second fingers held closely together, i.e., doubled. This makes them into a very effective probing instrument. Use them to perform circles and back-and-forths. Take your time; don't rush. Treat the entire area that surrounds your ear, paying particular attention to the tissue behind and below.

Are you finding thick tissue that becomes painful with gentle treatment? Move up into the scalp region. Let your fingers follow any pain or contracted areas. As you move outward, add multiple-finger movements.

Go back to the attachment and examine the sternomastoid itself. Move down and pincer it gently between thumb and bent forefinger as you go. Roll it gently, feeling for contracted, fibrotic or painful areas. Try some gentle single-finger circles, back-and-forths, and single-finger stationary presses. Move down to where the muscle attaches to the chest wall and examine and treat. Use single-finger, double-finger, and multiple-finger circles.

Explore and treat the tissues of your face. Let your fingers look for tight, contracted areas and for areas that cause any increase of your ear pain. For treatment of the upper back, refer to "Migraine and Muscle Contraction Headaches."

Examine and treat the skin overlying all the tissue areas you treated. Pay particular attention to the skin overlying the attachment of the sternomastoid. You will undoubtedly find it thickened and painful. Notice how thick the skin is as it blends into your ear. Use your thumb for skin ripples and circles. Treat thoroughly.

Dysfunctioning tissues that underlie ear pain may have been developing for a long period of time (years) before symptoms become apparent. Accordingly, these tissues may not respond quickly, and will require patient and diligent care to soften and normalize them so the pain will go away and stay away.

Emotional Pain (Associated with Panic Attacks, Sleep Disorders, Depression, Agoraphobia)

When an individual experiences emotional stress or trauma, body tissues tighten and contract and are, in effect, imprinted with that stress or trauma. Just as the tissues of the face reflect emotional stress, so do the tissues of the rest of the body. Once an emotional signal has been translated into a physical form, the imprinted physical component is now capable of recycling the signals, causing increasing emotional distress, as well as physical pain and physical dysfunction.

I have treated a few women who told me they had been sexually abused. Each experienced profound physical pain and dysfunction that was challenging and difficult to treat, in addition to their continuing emotional problems. I suspect that all victims of sexual abuse, and other severe emotional trauma, require soft tissue treatment to reverse and normalize the physical imprint (in addition to whatever psychotherapy they may be receiving) to achieve maximum healing. Attempting to treat a serious emotional problem without treating the physical component renders a disservice to the patient. The present-day psychiatric practitioner is apparently unaware of this.

There is a flip side to this. When an individual has been insulted by physical trauma, there frequently is a resulting emotional component, that is to say, an emotional overlay. In other words, both physical and emotional trauma can produce emotional symptoms. These can take the form of panic attacks, sleep disorder, depression, and agoraphobia. The patient in the following case history experienced all of these symptoms.

Case History

A woman in her fifties was referred for treatment of a severely painful shoulder. Her doctor informed me that because of "emotional problems" she was unable to leave her home, and I would have to treat her there. I phoned her and set up an appointment.

When I met with her, I learned that she had been injured in a car accident when she was five years old. She had also sustained very severe emotional trauma at an early age. Throughout the ensuing years, her body was plagued with pain and tightness and she suffered from severe headaches.

She also experienced emotional problems, depression, sleep disorder, and panic attacks, and she had recently been diagnosed as having agoraphobia (fear of being in a crowd or public place). She was aware that her physical and emotional problems were growing worse. Medications and psychological counseling had not helped. She lost her job because of these problems, and she said she was at the end of her strength.

When I examined her, I found that the tissues of her entire body were tight, contracted, fibrotic, and painful. Her shoulder was hurting, but so was the rest of her body. Her scalp, face, neck, and upper back were particularly tight and painful to light palpation.

After the first treatment, she said she felt more relaxed than she had for a long time. When I returned to give her a second treatment, she said that her body was still hurting but she had slept "a little better." As treatments continued, her physical pain and emotional problems became less severe. Two to three hours of fitful sleep was all she could attain when treatment started, but she gradually experienced deeper sleep for longer periods.

I treated her in two-hour sessions, three times a week for two weeks, then twice a week for two weeks. I was then able to reduce treatment to once a week for one month, then down to once every two weeks for a total of five months.

Because her problems were of such long duration—over fifty years—we were not able to achieve a complete recovery. However, when she was discharged at the end of five months, her condition had significantly improved. She could have five to six hours of refreshing sleep. Her emotional problems had lessened, and she was able to leave her house and start working again. She was extremely pleased with the results of the treatments.

Soft Tissue Manipulation Techniques

The areas of soft tissue dysfunction that are associated with emotional pain can occur anywhere in the body. Frequently, they are the same areas that generate headaches, that is, the scalp, face, neck, upper back, and chest. Refer to the headache section "Migraine and Muscle Contraction Headaches" for treatment suggestions. You may have to explore your body for other tissue areas that underlie your problem.

Fibromyalgia

Doctors coined the name fibromyalgia in the late 1970s to refer to a commonly occurring complaint: muscle pain. When patients suffering muscle pain (myalgia) are told by their doctors that they "have" fibromyalgia, they are impressed with the intelligence of their doctors. They don't realize their doctors have merely informed them in a fancy way that they have muscle pain, something they already knew. Fibromyalgia is another catchy name, in the long list of catchy names, doctors have invented to imply knowledge and impress their patients when knowledge is absent.

Doctors produce a diagnosis of fibromyalgia using a combination of two criteria as directed by The American College of Rheumatology Criteria for the Classification of Fibromyalgia:

1. *Pain throughout the body.* "Pain throughout the body" is not a useful basis of diagnosis.

2. *Pain in eleven of eighteen tender point sites.* This sounds scientific, but let's look a little closer. Medical literature tells us it is important that a tender point site cannot be tender, it must be painful. If it is tender, not painful when pressed upon, then it is not a countable tender point. How does the doctor know if a site

is either painful or tender? The patient tells him. It's sounding less scientific and more like subjective guesswork, isn't it? But wait, there's more.

Since the individual has pain all over, as expressed in criterion number one, it is likely that he will have pain wherever pressed. So doctors have come up with points "less likely to be painful" when pressed. They call these points "control points." If someone states they have pain in more than three control points, the doctor is inclined to feel she does not have fibromyalgia, even if she has those eleven of eighteen tender points, that is, painful points. What if a patient has only eight, nine, or ten of those painful tender point sites? What does she have?

Doctors do not understand that contracted skin, fascia, muscles, and ligaments can squeeze pain receptors, blood vessels, and nerves, thereby causing the symptoms of pain and fatigue to which they have affixed the empty word of fibromyalgia.

Doctors have given a name to another kind of point they press upon from time to time. They call this point a "trigger point." When busy pressing on a patient trying to differentiate painful, tender, and control points, the doctor has to be alert not to confuse any of those points with trigger points. Trigger points can be painful or tender, but doctors feel they are not related to what they call fibromyalgia. Still sounding scientific?

It is important that doctors press on all those points as they occur on all parts of their patients' bodies and with exactly the same amount of pressure as other doctors throughout the country, in order to make this a reproducible scientific examination technique. Doctors have decided that the reproducible pressure applied to all those points is the amount it takes to blanche a doctor's thumbnail. This must mean that all thumbnails, big, small, thick, thin, young, old, pointy, blunt—all blanche to the same degree when pressing on those various points.

The sad thing is that even if pressing on all those points leads to reproducible results, doctors still don't know what it is that causes those points to be tender or painful, or why their patients hurt all over and are so fatigued.

Doctors do not understand that contracted skin, fascia, muscles, and ligaments can squeeze pain receptors, blood vessels, and nerves, thereby causing the symptoms of pain and fatigue to which they have affixed the empty word of fibromyalgia.

It follows that since doctors do not understand the cause of what they call fibromyalgia, they do not know how to treat that cause. Because of their ignorance, they say fibromyalgia is incurable, and attempt to manage the symptoms with drugs, exercise, and diet. Individuals diagnosed as having fibromyalgia have called from time to time asking if I could help them. I told them I would need a doctor's prescription in order to examine and treat them. In all cases, their doctors refused to sign one. I have successfully treated individuals such as the patient mentioned in the chronic pain section, who would fit the current "criteria" of fibromyalgia.

Soft Tissue Manipulation Techniques

If you have been diagnosed as having fibromyalgia, you probably suffer from extensive areas of soft tissue dysfunction and have a lot of work ahead of you.

My treatment suggestions are the same that I offer for those classed as having "chronic pain."

Start by examining and treating your upper extremities. Refer to "Carpal Tunnel Syndrome" for soft tissue manipulation techniques. When the tissues of your arms and hands have become normalized and free of pain, you will be better able to treat other areas of your body that may be affected.

Frozen Shoulder

Frozen shoulder, a painful and disabling problem, is ill-defined and misunderstood by the medical community. The attention of doctors is focused at the point of the patient's complaint of pain: the shoulder joint. The problem, however, usually lies with contracted soft tissue well away from the joint. The medical profession is apparently unaware that pain perceived to be inside a joint is invariably radiated from dysfunctioning tissues outside the joint.

The upper extremity is connected to the torso primarily by muscles that are attached close to the shoulder joint. However, some of these muscles are large, and their torso attachment is far from the shoulder. The latissimus dorsi, for example, originates as far away as the pelvis.

If these muscles become contracted, the shoulder is not allowed to move freely. If severely contracted, they hold the shoulder tightly against the torso. The shoulder becomes "frozen." The problem is not with the shoulder joint, but with the contracted muscles attached to the shoulder joint.

The proper treatment for a "frozen shoulder," therefore, is to soften and normalize these muscles. When this is done, the shoulder moves freely again.

Case History 1

The patient I am about to discuss was treated very early in my career. Her case was pivotal in pointing me toward recognizing the global aspect of soft tissue dysfunction. She was a woman in her sixties, referred to me as a staff physical therapist.

She had a painfully frozen shoulder that had developed gradually over a two-year period, but the cause was unknown. Her shoulder had become excruciatingly painful three months before I saw her.

At that time, I knew little about soft tissue dysfunction. I had been taught that to treat a frozen shoulder, you applied moist heat to the shoulder joint, followed by ultrasound to the shoulder joint, followed by stretching of the shoulder joint. The stretching was performed both manually and with the aid of a "shoulder wheel," which produced an effect that must have been similar to what stretching a victim on the rack in the Middle Ages must have produced: intense and excruciating pain. I proceeded to practice what I had been taught, but when I attempted to stretch her shoulder, she cried out in pain. Being softhearted, I stopped.

The only thing I could think to do for her was to reach out and gently touch her painful shoulder to try to soothe it. It was a natural act of compassion rather than a treatment technique. However, this seemed to give her some relief, so I started to gently massage her shoulder and arm. She felt a little better at the end of the session, so another was scheduled.

This continued for several weeks. Gradually, her pain eased and the tightness around her shoulder softened. As those tissues softened, I became aware that tissues farther away from her shoulder were also tight, contracted, and painful. I began to work on those areas.

I found myself gradually working down her upper arm, forearm, and wrist. This was about two months into treatment. Finally, I was working on painful tissues in her hand and fingers, the last areas that needed treatment. Suddenly she remembered what had started the whole problem.

Two years earlier, a few months before she noticed pain in her shoulder, a purse had been snatched from her. In the struggle, two of her fingers had become injured and painful. The relationship between her injured fingers and her frozen shoulder had not occurred to her until I began to work on them and the remaining pain had jogged her memory.

It was only after, and because we had persistently tracked and released the tissue from her shoulder, down through her arm, forearm, hand, and fingers, that the connection was made. I figured the soft tissues had gradually tightened, somehow, from her injured finger on up to her shoulder.

The light was turned on. The global aspect and interconnectiveness of soft tissue dysfunction was revealed. A problem starting in a finger caused a problem in a shoulder. What this said to me was that a problem starting in any part of the body can cause a problem in any other part of the body, no matter how distant from each other the parts happen to be. Injure one part of the body, and eventually the entire body may become affected.

Case History 2

A woman in her early seventies came for treatment of a severely painful frozen shoulder. She had fractured her left humerus (the bone of the upper arm) six months earlier, and during the course of the healing, her shoulder had become frozen.

She had already received intensive physical therapy as prescribed by her doctor. The physical therapy consisted of hot packs, ultrasound, and stretching exercises to the shoulder joint. In addition, her doctor had injected cortisone into the shoulder joint. However, despite a long course of the above treatments, her shoulder had become increasingly painful and even more frozen.

She had heard of my work and had obtained a doctor's prescription that allowed me to treat her. Unfortunately, her doctor's prescription called for more of the same treatment already proven to be ineffective, namely, more hot packs, more ultrasound, and more stretching exercises. I called the doctor's office and was successful, after some difficulty, in having the order changed to "evaluate and treat," which allowed me to work in the manner I thought best.

When I examined the patient, I found that she had lost fifty per-cent of her shoulder movement. When she tried to move past the end point of her range of motion, she experienced severe pain at the shoulder. When I palpated her tissues, I found that the muscles and tissues outside her shoulder joint were tight, spasmed, contracted, and very painful to the touch. She was surprised that we were find-ing so many painful areas well away from her shoulder, some as far away as her lower back.

She responded well to treatment. By the end of her first two-hour treatment, she had gained an additional twenty percent of shoulder motion. I treated her daily for one week. Treatments were reduced to three times a week the following week, then to two times the next week. The next week was a one-time check-over.

At the time of discharge, four weeks after start of care, she had full range of motion, without any pain, and she was a very happy lady. A follow-up call two months later revealed she remained pain- and symptom-free; an additional call one year later, she was still pain- and symptom-free.

Of course I sent reports of my treatments to her doctor, but I received no response or inquiries from him as to what I had done for his patient that had caused her dramatic improvement.

Soft Tissue Manipulation Techniques

The primary areas of soft tissue dysfunction that contribute to so-called frozen shoulder are: (1) upper extremity; (2) chest; (3) upper back; and (4) mid to low back (latissimus dorsi muscle and associated tissues).

Treat the tissues of your upper extremity first. Refer to "Carpal Tunnel Syndrome" for soft tissue manipulation techniques.

Now treat your chest area. Refer to "Treating your chest" in the section titled "Migraine and Muscle Contraction Headaches."

Then treat your upper to lower back tissues. For soft tissue manipulation techniques of the upper back, refer to "Treating your neck and upper back" in "Migraine and Muscle Contraction Headaches." For the lower back, refer to "Back Pain."

Hip Pain and
Degenerative Joint Disease

Doctors believe that joints degenerate because of disease intrinsic to the joint itself; that is why they characterize the problem as a "joint disease." Doctors do not carefully examine the bodies of their patients and therefore do not understand that joint dysfunction is primarily caused by the prolonged stress of contracted body tissues *outside* the joint.

A joint is stressed when the tissues surrounding it become tight and contracted. If this stress continues over a protracted period, the structure of the joint begins to change, to degenerate. If this process is allowed to continue for years, the joint may become so damaged that it eventually has to be replaced with a plastic and metal one.

Fortunately, nature provides us with the early warning system of pain. Pain alerts the individual that something is wrong. The proper response of doctors would be to carefully examine the body to find what is causing the alarm signal of pain. Tight, contracted tissues would then be identified and treated, and the sensation of pain would go away, as well as the stress to the joint, which would remain healthy. Sadly, doctors do not heed the alarm signal of pain;

in fact, believe it or not, they actually attempt to kill it, and the dramatic growth of the mechanical-joint industry continues apace.

Case History

The histories of several patients I have treated over the years indicate that difficult birthings, and even not-so-difficult birthings, can contribute significantly to soft tissue dysfunction, which in turn causes the joints of the body to become dysfunctional. I can recall one woman in particular whose case illustrates this.

This woman noticed pain in her hips a few months after a difficult birth. As years went on, her knees also became painful. The pain gradually became severe and constant, and was accompanied by increasing tightness of her hips and knees. She was given pain medication, muscle relaxants, and cortisone injections, without any effect on either the pain or tightness.

I saw her thirty-four years after that difficult birth. As a matter of fact, it was my questioning about her early history that elicited her recollection about it and the ensuing pain and tightness. This had not been explored by any of the doctors who had treated her.

By the time soft tissue treatment was started, so many years following the onset of her problem, I was able to provide her with only limited improvement. The tissues on her right side were successfully released and became pain-free, but the joint structures of her left hip and knee were so damaged by the continued stress of contracted tissue for such a long period of time that I suggested she talk to her doctor about joint replacements.

This was done, and she became relatively pain-free. It is tragic that she had to suffer pain for so many years and eventually be subjected to drastic surgical joint replacement when timely soft tissue treatment likely would have prevented all her problems.

Soft Tissue Manipulation Techniques

Any joint in the body can be stressed by tight and contracted body tissues. If you suffer pain perceived to be coming from a joint, and intrinsic joint problems such as rheumatoid arthritis have been ruled out, and your doctor is talking about replacing your joint with a mechanical one, it would be wise to see if you can solve your problem by using soft tissue manipulation techniques. Refer to the appropriate symptom area that relates to where you are hurting. If you are experiencing hip pain, refer to "Back Pain." Also refer to treatment under "Knee Pain," as this structure is a frequent contributor to hip joint pain.

Knee Pain

Doctors attempt to treat knee pain with drugs, surgery, and the replacement of natural joints with mechanical ones. However, knee pain is frequently caused by contracted tissues *outside* the knee joint. The pain is *referred* to the inside of the joint. Although the sufferer can swear the pain is inside the joint, it is really radiated from exterior tissues.

The causative tissues are usually above the knee, in the thigh muscles and associated tissues. Less of a factor, although still a frequent component of knee pain, are the tissues below the joint.

A structure I call the "knee destroyer" runs down the outside of the thigh, from the hip to the knee. This is the tensor fascia lata. It is almost always involved in knee pain and dysfunction. The tensor fascia lata is a knee stabilizer. It is composed of a small muscle that starts at the hip and rapidly develops into a thick, strong band of fascia that attaches at the knee joint. But when this band becomes tight, contracted, and fibrotic, it causes severe pain and stresses the structures of the knee joint to which it is attached. When this stress continues over the course of years, the joint itself eventually becomes damaged.

Proper treatment is to soften and normalize the tight and contracted tissues that are radiating pain and causing stress to the knee joint. When this is done, the pain will go away and the knee joint will remain healthy.

Mechanical joint replacement is becoming increasingly popular these days. Indeed, mechanical joint replacement can be a blessing in eliminating the excruciating pain of severe joint dysfunction. The tragedy is that, often as not, the need for mechanical joint replacement can be entirely avoided, along with years of agonizing pain.

It takes a long period of time for the tight, contracted, and fibrotic tissues that surround a joint to eventually stress the structures of that joint to become so dysfunctional that it has to be replaced with one made of metal and plastic. During all those years, there are progressive alarm signals of pain that cry out for help. If doctors knew how to interpret those alarm signals and to properly respond to them, they could save their patients years of pain and the eventuality of drastic and mutilating surgery.

A structure I call the "knee destroyer" runs down the outside of the thigh, from the hip to the knee. It is almost always involved in knee pain and dysfunction. When this band becomes tight, contracted, and fibrotic, it causes severe pain and stresses the structures of the knee joint to which it is attached.

Case History 1

A woman was referred for treatment of a painful shoulder. When I chatted with her before treatment, I learned she was a retired surgical nurse. She had been forced to accept an early retirement fourteen years earlier because of a terribly painful right knee. Standing on hard floors for many years had apparently caused the knee problem. During all her years of retirement, she continued to suffer severe, agonizing pain.

I asked if anything had been done to help her knee pain. She said doctors had tried everything, but nothing had helped. Her orthopedic doctor told her the only thing that would end her pain was a mechanical knee replacement. She declined this procedure because of her experiences as a surgical nurse.

I told her there was a chance I might be able to help her painful knee. I called her doctor and received permission to try. We decided to split the treatment into two parts: first, we would work on her shoulder, then we would work on her knee.

Her shoulder responded quickly to treatment, well within an hour. When I palpated the tissues of her right leg, I found there was extensive tissue dysfunction, from her hip on down to her calf. Wherever I touched, I found tight, contracted, and fibrotic tissue. Particularly affected was her tensor fascia lata.

I worked on those tissues for an hour. When I felt they had loosened somewhat, I told her she could get down from the treatment table and we would see if she was any better. She got down and began to bend her knee back and forth. "This is a miracle," she said. "It doesn't hurt; it absolutely doesn't hurt."

She said she would be right back and hurriedly left the office. After a few moments, she returned. She had been *running* up and down the stairs. For years she had to hobble painfully up and down stairs with a stiff leg. She couldn't wait to get home and tell her son what had happened.

When she returned for a follow-up visit two days later, she reported she was continuing to feel fine, with no return of pain. When I palpated her tissues, I found there were still significant contracted areas.

I gave her two more treatments. The contracted areas were slow to respond, but she continued to remain pain-free. I suggested that, since she was doing so well, we try to see how she would do without further treatment, but to call me at the first sign of return of pain.

We kept in touch, and there was no return of pain. Two years after treatment, she called and told me she had something that would be of great interest to me.

She had been back to her orthopedic doctor for another matter, and in the course of the visit she asked if he recalled her painful knee and the necessity of a total knee replacement. He said he certainly did recall it. She then showed him how she could move her knee without any pain or discomfort. He asked, "Who *did* this to you?" She told him a "wonderful" (her word) physical therapist by the name of Bernard Schatz. I asked what he then said. Her reply was "nothing."

I last heard from her a few months later. She continued to feel fine. She was about to go on an ocean cruise and thought she would call to thank me for helping her and changing her life so much. Naturally, that made me feel wonderful.

By the way, I never heard from her orthopedic doctor. I thought he would have had enough professional interest to find out what I had done so he could use the information to help his other patients avoid having their natural joints replaced by mechanical ones, but I guess he didn't.

Case History 2

A dentist friend frequently complained of severe pain in his left knee. The pain started a few years earlier after he had injured his knee during martial arts practice. His complaints continued for over a year. I told him I would be glad to take a look and see if there was something I could do to help. He said no, his knee had already been examined by an orthopedic doctor, and the only thing that could help was surgery.

He continued to decline my offer to see if there was anything I could do. His thinking was that the pain was coming from inside the knee joint, and there was nothing I could do to help a problem coming from *inside* the knee by working on the tissues *outside*. He felt the only thing that could possibly help him was surgical intervention, which he wanted to avoid as long as possible.

I told him that frequently when someone is certain pain is coming from within a joint, it actually is being *referred* from outside the joint. He remained firm in his conviction that the problem was dysfunction inside the knee.

One day, however, he called to say his knee was so excruciatingly painful that he was willing to see if there was something I could do to help him, even if just a little. I told him to get a doctor's prescription and I would see him.

When I examined him, I found the tissues of his thigh from his hip down were contracted. His tissues responded well. I could feel

A primary cause of knee pain and dysfunction is the "Knee Destroyer" (tensor fascia lata) that runs down the outer thigh. After years of gradual tightening and pain, it deranges the knee joint to such an extent that the joint has to be replaced with a metal and plastic one. Timely soft tissue work avoids this drastic and mutilating surgery.

them soften as I worked on them. After an hour, they had softened appreciably. I told him he could get off the treatment table and see how his knee felt. He got down, put some weight on his leg, bent his knee, walked around the office, and announced that he had no pain whatsoever. That was eight years ago. His knee has remained pain-free since that one treatment.

Case History 3

A woman in her sixties called to see if I could help her. She had received an artificial knee joint three months earlier but continued to experience severe knee pain. She complained to the surgeon who had performed the joint replacement, but he had dismissed her complaints of pain.

When I examined her, I found that the tissues above her knee were swollen and painful to light touch. I treated them gently, and when the swelling subsided, contracted tissues were revealed. These responded to treatment, and in one month she was discharged, pain-free.

She was pleased with the results of treatment, and did not question the need for her joint replacement, or how it could be that she was able to experience pain in a knee joint that was now a mechanical one. I left those matters undiscussed.

Soft Tissue Manipulation Techniques

Knee pain is primarily caused by: (1) dysfunction above the knee (thigh muscles and associated tissues), and (2) dysfunction below the knee (muscles and associated tissues of the calf and shin). Dysfunctioning tissues in the lower back, hip, and foot may be contributing factors of knee pain. If pain persists after thorough treatment of primary areas, review soft tissue manipulation techniques of these tissues.

Treatment of thigh muscles and associated tissues. You need to purchase a foot stool (inexpensive plastic ones are available). Get yourself into a comfortable sitting position. Let us assume your right knee is the painful one. Place some towels under your thigh and a pillow on the stool. Put your right foot on the pillow and position the stool away from you until your knee is as straight as comfort will allow. This will slacken the portion of thigh tissues you will be treating first.

Place your hand on your thigh. That is where you will start treatment: on the front of your thigh (the top as you look down on it). Apply some lotion. Grasp the large bulk of muscle there between your thumb and fingers. See how it starts up at your hip and funnels down to your kneecap. This is the muscle that straightens your knee. Get acquainted with it and its associated tissues. Take your time. Try thumb sweeps over the skin. Try to ripple the skin. Do you find thickened and painful areas? These are indicators of dysfunctioning tissues underneath. Note where they are; they will have to be softened and normalized. This is a first get-acquainted session, so you will be discovering many things. Don't worry about getting everything treated this first time.

With your fingers held together, make deeper sweeps up and down from hip to knee. Do you find thickened, painful lumps? Explore them with single- and multiple-finger circles and nudges. Are you finding areas that become painful as you gently explore them? These are hidden pain areas, where pain has been stored up for a long period of time. They will have to be released and normalized—more than one session will be required.

All of these dysfunctioning areas—and the ones that remain to be discovered—are contributors to your knee pain.

Explore your kneecap. Use thumb and forefinger nudges, circles, and side-to-sides. Go entirely around the kneecap. Keep looking for tight, painful areas. Then use both hands, with fingers held close together, to perform circles, nudges, and side-to-sides around your kneecap.

Using both your hands, continue those movements to explore the bony ridges on both sides of your knee. You will likely find hard, painful tissue adherent to those bony ridges. These have to be softened and their pain released.

Apply lotion to the outside of your thigh. Starting at the knee, explore upward toward your hip with multiple-finger circles. You will notice a thick, tough band that runs the entire length of your thigh. This is the tensor fascia lata, although I call it the Knee Destroyer. Its job is to stabilize the hip and knee when you stand and walk about. This demanding assignment stresses it, and, as the years pass, it may become severely dysfunctional. With the passage of time, it progressively tightens, causing knee pain. If it is not treated in a timely fashion, derangement of the knee joint is likely. Prolonged stress of a tight tensor fascia lata may also cause derangement of the hip joint.

The tensor fascia lata and the tissues adjoining it require thorough treatment. Grasp the tissues on the right side of your thigh between thumb and fingers. Gently squeeze those tissues, from knee up to hip; then down, from hip to knee. Repeat several times. This will begin the softening process. (When you are up at the hip area, feel free to move out and explore your gluteal tissues. Keep looking for tight, contracted, painful tissues wherever you find them. Let your fingers explore freely. Keep in mind that *all parts* of your body are interconnected.)

Now try to ripple your skin using thumb to finger sweeps (thumb on top of thigh, fingers underneath). Notice how thick, adherent, and painful the skin is as you pass over the tensor fascia lata. Are you surprised at the amount of pain you are finding there? Are you surprised that you have walked around with all that pain for years, blissfully unaware of what had happened to your body?

Continue with several of these sweeps. With doubled fingers, gently explore the tensor fascia lata with circles, nudges, and side-to-sides. There can be considerable hidden pain associated with the tensor fascia lata. Be prepared to experience tenderness following even gentle treatment. Post-treatment tenderness is temporary. It lessens with succeeding treatments. Usually, with just a few treatments you will no longer experience any pain, although tissue tightness may linger.

By this time you have likely awakened considerable hidden pain, so move on to your inner thigh tissues. Apply lotion at the uppermost portion of your inner thigh. You will likely find considerable hidden pain here. Indeed, gentle exploration frequently elicits an excruciating amount of pain—so be very gentle. Again, you may wonder how it was possible for you to live with so much pain and yet be unaware of it until you gently explored. Use gentle thumb and finger sweeps across the skin, proceeding down to the knee. Explore the deeper inner thigh tissues using manipulation movements already described. Use your thumb to explore tissues close to your knee.

You will now treat the remaining thigh tissues, those at the back of your thigh (underneath as you sit). Use fingers of both hands to perform circles and nudges for these tissues. Now go back over all treated areas with waves.

You are not yet finished with the treatment of your thigh tissues. Remember how earlier in the book I mentioned that I explore and treat patients in *all* positions? This is particularly important for treatment of the thigh. So, after treating in the sitting position, go back over those tissues while lying on your right side and left side. Every position reveals additional important information and the ability to provide effective treatment.

It is likely you were not able to explore all thigh tissues in even one position in one treatment session, particularly the first session. You may well have been so interested in what you found that just a very small area was explored and treated. Go at your own pace. It is all interesting and exciting, isn't it!

Treatment of calf and shin tissues. Let's start with your calf. Cross your legs so that your right ankle rests on your left knee. This will allow good treatment access to your inner and posterior calf. Using both hands, perform thumb sweeps across your entire calf. Look for tight, painful skin areas. Notice how the skin becomes crinkly, adherent, and painful as you approach your shin. This area will require patient and diligent treatment.

Now place the fingers of your left hand under your calf, so they move your calf opposite to how gravity is causing it to sag. While your left hand continues to support your calf, use your right thumb to perform circles and nudges throughout your entire calf.

Go slowly. You will find extensive areas of knots and contracted/spasmed tissues. Your calf muscle has rendered you an enormous amount of work during its lifetime. Every time you took a step, it lifted your entire body weight! But in the course of this lifetime of work, it has become dysfunctional. You now have an opportunity to say "thank you" to it.

As you work on your calf and discover how much of it has become infiltrated with thick, contracted, fibrotic tissue, you will realize how limited and ineffective are the crude stretchings that doctors and their operatives offer. Only careful and thorough soft tissue treatments are able to normalize severe soft tissue dysfunction.

To work on the outside of your calf, put an additional pillow or two on the stool. When you uncross your legs and place your right foot on this higher elevation, you will be better able to reach the tissues of your outer calf. Perform skin sweeps with your thumb. Multiple-finger circles and nudges are effective for deeper tissues of this portion of your calf.

While your leg is in this position, you will be able to extend treatment to the tissues of your shin. With both your hands, perform thumb sweeps over the entirety of your shin. You will undoubtedly notice how tightly drawn your skin is, and when you perform multiple-finger circles on the deeper shin tissues, you will realize how tight and contracted those tissues have become.

Your shin muscle also has performed a lifetime of noble work for you. Each time you took a step, it lifted your foot clear off the ground so you would not stumble. It is a small muscle and its task is a challenging one. The daily lifting of your foot (hundreds and hundreds of times each day for years) caused it to become tight, contracted, and fibrotic. In the future, when healthcare is more responsive to a patient's real needs, you will receive periodic treatments that will prevent your muscles from becoming dysfunctional and contributing to knee pain. But now you will have to provide restorative treatment. Your shin tissues and your calf tissues will require extensive treatment, but it will be well worth it when they are soft, supple, and no longer contribute to your knee pain.

Logger's Hand

Hands can be abused by all sorts of trauma. As a case in point, I present the following.

Case History

I coined the term "logger's hand" to describe a patient I treated a few years ago. The gentleman was in his mid-forties and had been a logger since his mid-teens. For thirty years, he had worked in all extremes of weather and had received numerous injuries, including fractures to his hands and arms. He had pulled heavy log chains with his bare hands, had used all kinds of heavy equipment that injured his hands, and had generally abused his hands to an extent I have not observed before or since.

The result was a pair of hands that were almost completely non-functional. He was unable to work as a logger because he could not hold or use a chain saw or any other logging equipment. Most sadly, he had a three-year-old, and he told me, with tears in his eyes, that he was so helpless he could not even button the child's clothing. He was reluctant to try my treatments but came because a friend who knew of my work had insisted.

His hands and fingers were thick, stiff, and painful. He could bend his fingers only very slightly. He held his hands with his fingers outstretched. The tissues of the rest of his upper extremities were also affected, but not nearly so much as his hands.

At the beginning of the first visit, he held out his hands and said, "There ain't no way that anybody can help these-here hands." After the first treatment was over, however, he had to admit that his fingers did seem to be a "little looser," and his hands did feel a "little better."

We continued treatment twice a week for eight weeks. At the end of this time, he had regained full use of his hands, although some mid-palm tightness remained. He had resumed full-time work as a logger and was able to button his child's clothing. He was discharged, happy and pleased.

Soft Tissue Manipulation Techniques

For appropriate soft tissue manipulation techniques, refer to "Carpal Tunnel Syndrome."

Migraine and Muscle Contraction Headaches

Doctors contend there are primarily two kinds of head pain, which they name migraine and muscle contraction headaches. Doctors admit they do not know what causes migraines but think they are associated somehow with vascular dysfunction of a vague and ill-defined nature. Doctors consider migraine to be incurable.

Doctors think muscle contraction headache, sometimes called tension headache, is caused by contracted or tense muscles. They are getting a little closer here, but their analysis is so simplistic that any treatment value is lost. Doctors consider migraine and muscle contraction headaches to be unrelated. Unable to treat the cause, they attempt to "manage" the pain of all headaches with drugs.

Several years ago, I became aware of the relationship of head pain to soft tissue dysfunction. When I treated patients for upper back problems, I noted that they frequently stated they also suffered from headaches. Some had been diagnosed as having migraine headaches, others as having muscle contraction headaches. The interesting thing was that both types of headaches became milder and less frequent as the tight and contracted tissues of their backs softened and became pain-free.

As I gained experience, I refined my ability to identify and treat the tissues that cause headaches. I now know it is extremely important to examine the scalp, face, neck, and upper chest, as well as the back, for tight, contracted, and fibrotic areas. When these are found and palpated, a headache will frequently be elicited, which confirms the relationship of soft tissue dysfunction and the headache symptom. Another frequent response to this treatment is this: "Oh, that's just where I get my headache!"

I now know it is extremely important to examine the scalp, face, neck, and upper chest, as well as the back, for tight, contracted, and fibrotic areas. When these are found and palpated, a headache will frequently be elicited, which confirms the relationship of soft tissue dysfunction and the headache symptom.

It is necessary to treat, reverse, and normalize all dysfunctioning tissues found to contribute to your headache symptoms for you to become free of pain and stay free of pain, as follows:

Scalp. Your scalp is not just a piece of skin stretched over the skull to provide a foundation for hair to grow out of. It contains an extensive network of stress-receiving, stress-storing, and stress-triggering tissues. When these become tight, contracted, and fibrotic, they send out alarm signals of pain that are called migraine and muscle contraction headaches.

Face. Tissues of your face should be soft, supple, and free of pain. Tissues underlying the skin at the nasal sinuses should not be hard, thick, or painful, nor should the tissues around your eyes. When skin under the jaw line is gently moved between the thumb and fingers, it should not feel lumpy or painful. These are all signs of soft tissue dysfunction that likely contribute to your headache.

Tissues of the face receive, absorb, and store messages of internal and external stress. Creases form, with fibrotic tissue underlying each crease. The greater the accumulation of stress, the thicker the underlying layer of fibrotic tissue, and the deeper the crease. As this process continues year after year, more and more tissue dysfunction develops, and more and more hidden pain is stored away.

The face is the primary area of the body that expresses our emotions. In order to express emotions, its tissues must be strong receivers of emotional messages, many of which are stressful in nature. Look at photographs of Abraham Lincoln taken at different times as the Civil War progressed. You can see how the tissues of his face changed, how they became tight, contracted, and fibrotic.

Constantly bombarded by these messages, the tissues of the face become part of a stress loop, later sending stress messages back out to the body. So one might say that the individual causes his face to become stressed. On the other hand, the face causes the individual to become stressed.

Your face should be treated, not only to improve your appearance and to normalize painful areas, but also to reduce the stress signals that are being sent out so you can become fully healthy again. Just as with other areas of your body, the tissues of your face will respond to proper treatment by becoming soft and supple. You will be astonished how relaxed and stress-free you become after the tissues of your face are properly treated and released, and your headaches go away.

Neck: The tissues of your neck should be soft and supple. The two bands of muscles at the front of the neck (sternomastoids) and their associated tissues should not be hard or painful to palpation, particularly at their upper ends where they attach behind the ears. All the tissues of the neck (front, sides, and back) should be carefully examined for areas of dysfunction. They are frequently headache generators and must be normalized if pain-free health is to be achieved.

Back: The tissues of your back, particularly the upper back, are important contributors of head pain. The trapezius muscle is almost always involved. Its job is to hold your head upright; therefore, it is in a state of constant tension whenever you sit, stand, or walk about. The only time it has to rest is when you lie down. This constant tension causes the muscle to become extremely tight, contracted, and fibrotic (i.e., dysfunctional). The signals of distress it sends out adds to your headache.

Chest: The pectoral muscles and their associated tissues, located at your chest, can be contributors of head pain. They also have to be examined and, if found to be dysfunctional, must be treated, if freedom from headaches is to be achieved.

Case History 1

I was speaking with a young neurology resident at a teaching hospital. In the course of our conversation, I mentioned that I treated migraine patients. I told her of some of my experiences and explained my treatment rationale. She became very interested and said that she and her associates would keep me busy treating migraine patients, as there was a long list of them in her department and they were suffering severe pain and not being helped.

The resident said that just that morning she had examined a twenty-six-year-old woman who had suffered migraines for nine years. She experienced severe migraines daily, and every few days was so incapacitated by a particularly excruciating migraine that she had to go to an emergency room for injections of medication. The woman told her that these episodes of increased pain, accompanied by nausea and vomiting, were nightmarish.

The patient had just returned from an extensive workup at a new multimillion-dollar headache center, where the doctors there told her the drugs she was taking were appropriate, and that nothing more could be done to reduce the severity or frequency of her migraines.

The neurology resident said she would immediately refer this woman for treatment and that numerous referrals from the doctors in her unit would soon follow. I told her to please limit the referrals to not more than ten. This would allow me the time necessary to treat each one on a quality basis.

The young woman did call, and we started treatment the next day. When I examined her, I found the tissues of her scalp, neck, upper back, and chest to be severely contracted. Particularly affected were the tissues of her scalp and neck. Her scalp was drawn tight as a drum and was intensely painful to the lightest touch.

I treated her daily in two-hour sessions. The first treatments were stormy, because even lightly touching the affected areas elicited a headache. But she continued to return for further treatment for two reasons: one, the very fact that touching the tight, contracted tissue caused a headache demonstrated that the tight, contracted tissue was the underlying cause of her headaches; and two, after each treatment she felt her body becoming looser.

After the first few treatments, the reactions became milder, and she noticed that between treatments her headaches were less severe and less frequent. After three weeks, she reported that she had gone two days without a headache. She considered this to be a miracle.

I continued to treat her daily for three months. During this time, her tissues progressively softened, and, although there were days when she still experienced a severe headache, their intensity and frequency diminished. She no longer had to suffer the night-mare of emergency-room visits.

The next two months brought continued improvement. Most days were completely headache-free. Occasionally, she experienced a mild headache at infrequent intervals. These were usually aborted by using a small microcurrent unit I had given her. At this time, her entire quality of life had changed, and she was a different person.

I sent reports to the neurology department and to the resident who had made the referral, describing how the patient was improv-ing, but I received no reply from them. Nor did I receive any more referrals of the "many migraine patients that were not being helped" by the conventional approaches.

The doctors could see her dramatic improvement, and could hear her comments describing her improvement, when she reported for rechecks to their department. Yet, to my puzzlement, no more migraine sufferers were referred to me. One day, as I was chatting with my patient, I mentioned my puzzlement to her.

"How naive you are, Bernard. Don't you understand what hap-pened? When the resident reported to her chief that she had referred me to you, she was probably reprimanded and told, 'We do the migraine patients here, we do not refer them out.'"

I would have wanted to continue to treat this patient to get her completely free of pain, but she moved away from the area. I received a letter from her two years later saying that she was con-tinuing to do well with no return of prior symptoms. It is unfortu-nate that this young woman had to endure nine nightmarish years when appropriate treatment early on could probably have prevented any headaches from developing.

Case History 2

A young woman was referred to me because of severe, excruciating headaches that had been occurring on a daily basis for over a year. The headaches started at the back of her head, then went over her scalp, and ended in agonizing pain behind her eyes. Her doctor had diagnosed them as muscle contraction headaches. She described the pain as "terrible" and "unbearable." The pain medications and muscle relaxants her doctor had given her had not helped, and she told me she was ready for God to take her.

When I examined her, I found that the tissues of her upper back, neck, and scalp were severely contracted, and the overlying skin was drawn tight and adherent to the underlying tissues. All these tissues were extremely tender to mild palpation. She tolerated only the mildest of treatment for the first week. Gradually, as her tissues loosened and softened, she tolerated more treatment, and her headaches lessened in intensity and frequency.

At the end of a month, she no longer experienced any headaches. I continued treatment at decreasing frequency for two

Primary areas that cause headaches

more months, until I could no longer feel any tight or contracted tissues, and then discharged her.

Here was a case that doctors had called a muscle contraction headache, but that was a misdiagnosis. Her skin, muscles, and fascia were tight, thick, and fibrotic. The muscles were not contracted in the common sense, and there is no pain medication or muscle relaxant in the world that could have reversed and normalized this woman's problem.

Soft Tissue Manipulation Techniques

Important areas to be treated include (1) scalp, (2) face, (3) neck, (4) upper back, and (5) chest.

Other body areas may be affected, but the above are almost always involved. Start your treatment lying face up and support your head comfortably, with as many pillows as needed.

Treating your scalp. Start your headache treatment at the scalp. The scalp is the one and only area where lotion should not be used. I tried it once. Trust me, it doesn't work. Your hair itself will act as a sort of "lubricant." However, if part of your scalp is hair deficient, you can use lotion there.

Take your time and get acquainted with your scalp. Slip one hand behind your head so the palm supports the back of your head. This will free your thumb and fingers to explore and treat. Use your fingertips, all of them at the same time, to make exploratory circles. Start with small circles. Enlarge the circles. Try slow circles, then faster ones. Try back-and-forths with all your fingers. Now use your forefinger as the primary probe. As you continue with your scalp (and other tissue area) explorations, try the different finger configurations explained in the glossary. Refer to it from time to time for manipulation suggestions; try variations of pressure. Press firmly. Press lightly.

Alternate your right and left examining hands frequently so they do not get fatigued. As you explore the various areas of your scalp, move the supporting palm accordingly: from the back of your head, to the right side, left side, to the front.

The purpose of all this is to find and soften tight, painful areas. Scalp dysfunction can take various forms. Have your fingers look for very small, hard, painful, fibrotic knots. Move your fingers carefully, or you may miss some. When you find one, stay with it. If it is very painful, lighten your touch, but stay with it. Try very small back-and-forths, circles, or stationary probes on that painful, hard knot. You will likely feel the pain ease and disappear. If you then move off the area, you won't be able to find the knot again. It will no longer be there.

Something may happen when you press on that knot: It may trigger a headache. It seems ironic, to try to help yourself and then cause a headache. It is like pressing a "headache button." The only way you can soften that button and make it go away, so it will eventually cease causing headaches, is to touch it. This is anguishing, to cause pain in order to make it go away, yet it is curative.

It would have been far better if this had been properly treated years earlier, before things became so severe. But unfortunately this was not done, and you now have no choice but to deal with your present reality. You must work on that knot until it goes away, so lighten your touch to the weight of a feather. It may be that it is so established that it will not soften in one treatment; it may take several treatments to soften and normalize it. If so, that is what you will have to do. Be assured that persistence and coaxing will pay off.

Something else may happen when you press on that knot. You may, for example, feel pain generated at a distant point, at your shoulder or chest. This is one of those TCF loops (tight, contracted, fibrotic) mentioned earlier in this book. When this happens, I suggest that you also work on the shoulder or chest. Chances are you will then feel pain generated back up to your scalp. Both areas have to be normalized.

Another form of scalp dysfunction is a band of tight, contracted tissue. A pair can usually be found running from the forehead backward to where the skull starts curving down, bordering the area where men frequently are bald. These can be stubborn and resistant to softening. Double-finger back-and-forths are helpful here. Be patient and persistent. More than one session will probably be required.

Yet another configuration of dysfunction is a broad area of tight tissue just above and behind each ear, near where the sternomastoid muscle attaches. These can be extremely tender and painful. Try gentle circles, back-and-forths, and stationary presses. It is important to resolve these areas. (Refer to the section "Ear Pain" for detailed instructions.)

Work back and to the sides, toward your temples. You undoubtedly will find severely thickened and tender tissue there—this is where the temporomandibular muscle attaches, an important area.

When you go back as far as you can before you run into the pillows supporting your head, turn your head to one side so you can reach the back of your scalp. This will get you to your occipital area, where your posterior neck muscles attach. This area is of extreme importance. Treat it carefully and thoroughly with firm thumb and finger circles. Then turn to the other side and treat the remaining area of scalp tissue.

When all areas have been treated, go back and give a nice, light "once-over" to tie everything together. Use all fingers of both hands in broad circular sweeps. When you do this, think of getting the circulation going all through your scalp.

You can easily have spent two hours in your scalp exploration and treatment. I hope you found it interesting, and that you now realize your scalp is an area of great complexity and importance.

Treating your face. After you treat your scalp, I suggest you move down to your face. Now you will need the lotion and a cup of warm water. The forehead is a good place to start. Apply a small amount of lotion there. Place the thumb of your examining hand under your cheekbone. That will give you leverage and control when your fingers are placed on your forehead. Begin by examining some skin creases. Try small circles on a crease; be gentle. Then try stationary and side-to-side presses. Do you feel pain deep in the crease? Does it trigger pain to another area of your face? Up to your scalp? Behind an eye? Is it associated with your headaches?

Move along the entire length of the crease. Take your time. If the lotion dries out, apply a bit more, or perhaps a drop or two of water. If you like the feel of friction when you work on the crease, apply additional lotion later. Thoroughly explore the crease, then move on to another crease.

Perhaps you are curious because your fingers found an area of hardened skin, so explore that area of skin. Does it become painful after a moment or two of gentle palpation? Does it trigger pain elsewhere? Is it associated with your headaches? Gently squeeze that area of skin. Can you ripple it? Is it adherent to the tissues underneath? Does it become more painful as you work with it? Does it begin to soften as you work with it? Does the pain lessen?

Don't forget to change hands from time to time so they don't get tired.

Try some large sweeps across your entire forehead. Sweep across all your forehead creases. Try some large back-and-forths with all your fingers. Whenever you find something interesting (painful, hard, adherent, thick), pause and work on it. Now concentrate on the area just above your eyebrows. Try a variety of movements. Move down to the eyebrows proper.

Don't rush; always take your time. Go wherever your fingers lead you. Learn to trust your fingers.

Explore your entire forehead, up to your scalp line and down to the bridge of your nose. The tissue at the bridge of your nose can be an important component of headache production. Try pincering it firmly with a static hold. Do you feel pain developing? Does it radiate to your eyes? To your head? Is it associated with your headaches?

Move out to the sides of your forehead, to your temples. You will be forgiven if you intrude back onto your scalp, where your temporomandibular muscle attaches, for another going-over there.

Now place a forefinger at each depression just behind the ridge at the outer edge of your eyes. Move your forefingers in small, firm circles. Any pain there? If you find some (you likely will), follow it. Does it go back up to your forehead? Any association with your headaches? Do you find thick, contracted tissues? Will these tissues need further treatment?

Place some lotion on your face on either side of your nose (the sort of triangle between your nose and your cheekbones). Explore these areas carefully with back-and-forths and circles. Do they feel thickened and tight? Is one side thicker than the other? Any pain there? Any association with your headache? When you press on these, is a headache generated? These are your sinus areas. It is very likely they will need continued care before they become softened, normalized, and healthy. (Refer to the sections titled "Sinus Headache" and "Sinus Pain" for more detailed instructions.)

Work down the tissues overlying your jaws. It is likely these tissues are dysfunctional and important pain generators. Brace your thumb on the underside of your jaw. This will give your exploring fingers leverage and control. Thoroughly investigate and treat these tissues with the variety of techniques you are now getting familiar with.

Check the tissues that are closely attached to your jawbone. Follow its entire length. Look for hard, wirelike, adherent formations toward the front of the jaw. Run your thumb back and forth. Any pain in these? (Refer to "TMJ Pain" for detailed instructions on treating jaw tissues.)

You have now explored and treated your face and scalp. Did you find areas that are associated with your headache? I would be surprised if you didn't. Are you surprised at what you found? Were your explorations interesting? Do you feel you know more about your body? Your headaches?

You are now ready to proceed with your headache treatment.

Treating your neck and upper back. Tissues of your neck are a continuation of tissues of your trunk. I am speaking of the major neck muscles: the pair of sternomastoids in the front, and the trapezius in the back. It is important to treat these muscles thoroughly, particularly where they attach to the head.

The sternomastoids are the two long, narrow muscles that begin at the upper chest, run up the front of your neck, and attach just behind your ears. The trapezius is the broad, thick muscle of your upper back; it attaches to the bumps at the back of your head. It is the muscle that gets increasingly tight and painful as the day goes on.

I suggest you treat your sternomastoids first. (Please note that whenever muscles are mentioned, their associated skin and fascia must also be treated.)

Lie face up, with your head on extra pillows, so it is tilted forward. This will put some slack in your sternomastoids and make it easier for you to work on them. Start at the middle of either the right or left muscle. Let us say you start with the one on your right.

Grasp it between your thumb and the knuckle of your forefinger and gently roll it back and forth. This will likely elicit some level of discomfort, so be very gentle. Do this for a few seconds, then move downward toward your trunk. Continue treating until you reach the part that is attached to your collarbone (that's the cleido part of sternocleidomastoid). Work the collarbone attachment with circles, back-and-forths, and double-finger nudges. You will likely find painful tissue there.

Continue along your collarbone toward the center of your chest, toward your sternum (the sterno part of the name). Work this area carefully, again with circles, back-and-forths, and double-finger nudges.

Turn your head to the right so you are looking toward your right shoulder. This will slacken the muscle where it attaches to the bump behind the ear, the mastoid process, an important headache area. Go back to the middle of the muscle and work up to where it is firmly attached to your head, where you can't move it anymore. Probe this area thoroughly with your fore and middle fingers held together. Feel free to go back up into your scalp if interesting things draw you there. Use your thumb to explore and treat. I feel certain you will find significant pain areas here. Do you?

When you have explored this sternomastoid thoroughly, treat the other one in a similar manner. Don't forget to turn your head to the left when you work on its mastoid attachment.

You will now treat your trapezius. It may not seem feasible to treat tissues at the back of your neck and down between your shoulders, but it can be done. I know, because I have treated myself in these areas.

Arrange the pillows so your head is tilted backward, giving the muscle some slack. Remember, the trapezius is responsible for keeping your head upright throughout the day. It works continuously, never relaxing, and is truly a stressed and dysfunctional muscle. Accordingly, it underlies many pain problems, including headaches. Persistence and patience are required to normalize it.

The palm of your examining hand is behind your head. Place your fingers on one side of the attachment of the trapezius, and your thumb on the other. Use your thumb to make small, firm circles where the muscle attaches. This may lead you back into the scalp. Continue making firm circles; do the same with the fingers. Thoroughly examine the attachment area. Follow painful, thick tissues, even if this leads you away from the trapezius.

After you explore these, make your way back to the attachment. Work slowly. Undoubtedly, you will find an abundance of things to work on. Change hands from time to time to avoid fatigue. Gently pincer the muscle below the attachment between your thumb and forefinger. Coax it with push-pulls, then little circles. Try gentle kneading movements. Work down two or three inches, to where the muscle begins to widen. Now, with your right hand, reach around your front toward the back of your left shoulder. You will rest your palm on your collarbone, allowing your thumb and fingers free to explore the trapezius.

Because you are lying on your back, your trapezius will be as relaxed as possible. Press upward into the muscle with all your fingers held close together. Use soothing circles. Do you get the feeling that your careworn trapezius is saying, "Ah, relief at last"? No doubt you will find tight, contracted, and fibrotic areas throughout. Explore and soothe. Use your thumb to make circles into the muscle. Pincer it between thumb and fingers and perform push-pulls. Don't forget to treat the skin overlying your trapezius.

Work down to your shoulder blade. I'll wager you find a lot of hidden pain there. Treat this area thoroughly. Treat the portion of the trapezius that attaches to your spinal column; circle each vertebrae; work down as far as you can reach. Don't rush; let your tissues enjoy their long-neglected bliss. When you have done this to your tissues' satisfaction, use your left hand to treat your right trapezius. Although your trapezius will require patient and persistent treatment, your efforts will be rewarded when it no longer causes your headaches.

Treating your chest. Apply some lotion to the inner side of your shoulder at the level of your collarbone. Use small single- and multiple-finger circles and move horizontally, just under your collarbone, toward the center of your chest to the sternum.

Enlarge the circles until they sweep the area enclosed by an imaginary line from the shoulder joint to the top of the sternum, down the sternum, out to the rib cage, then back up to the shoulder joint. This will form a rectangle known as the chest rectangle.

Explore and treat the tissues attached to the collarbone, using all your fingers to sweep horizontally, then try small multiple-finger circles for the same tissues. Treat the skin with thumb ripples. When you come to where the sternomastoids are attached, feel free to re-explore those muscles and their associated tissues.

Carefully explore down the sternum using multiple-finger circles and back-and-forths. When you come to the bottom of the sternum, continue the multiple-finger circles out to where you can feel your ribs.

Continue upward toward the original starting point of the shoulder joint. The tissue along this rim of the chest rectangle is the outer edge of the pectoral muscle. When treating this area of the right pectoral, use your left hand. Place the palm of your hand on your chest. Position your thumb on the front of the edge of the muscle with your fingers curled around and behind it. Pincer the muscle between thumb and fingers. Use your index finger to perform circles upward into the muscle.

Every cubic centimeter of dysfunctional tissue has to be treated and normalized if full health is to be attained. Keep at it. It takes work and dedication. But it will be worth all the effort when your headaches are gone and your body feels wonderful again.

Examine and treat in this manner along the entire edge of the muscle. When you reach the shoulder joint, bring your fingers to the front and use multiple-finger circles and thumb sweeps. Continue with single- and double-finger movements. Be very gentle here, because it is an area that can contain severe hidden pain. Use plenty of lotion diluted with water so your fingers and thumb can slip easily over your skin. You may be surprised how much pain you find here, so go slowly. You may be further surprised that in just a few days it is likely you will no longer find any pain there; the area will be healed. Treat the opposite side in a similar manner.

Now you have finished treating the tissues that are the primary headache generators. Did you notice how quickly the time went?

Every cubic centimeter of dysfunctional tissue has to be treated and normalized if full health is to be attained. Keep at it. It takes work and dedication. But it will be worth all the effort when your headaches are gone and your body feels wonderful again.

Muscle Weakness

When muscles become infiltrated with fibrotic tissue, they lose their elasticity and ability to perform efficiently. They become weak. Exercise does not improve this kind of weakness, even though doctors prescribe it for this condition. Many patients who complain of increasing weakness of their arms, hands, and fingers are put on exercise programs by their doctors in an attempt to get them stronger. Yet the more they exercise, the weaker they become.

Patients are recycled year after year through "strengthening" programs, only to grow weaker. These individuals come to me, not for more strengthening, but because of the severe pain they are experiencing. I learn of their weakness when I examine them. Here is the interesting thing: When I treat and reverse the tight, fibrotic tissue that causes their pain, their strength increases, frequently quite dramatically, at the very first treatment. It is a wonderful experience to have someone come for a treatment experiencing severe pain and weakness, and have them leave with little or no pain and normal, or almost normal, strength.

In these cases, their muscles were weaker because they were bound down by tight, fibrotic tissue—the same tight, fibrotic tissue that was causing the pain that brought them to me. When I softened and released the fibrotic tissue, their muscles were able to function properly, and their strength returned. The exercise programs they were on only stimulated the production of more fibrotic tissue; they were not curative.

Case History

A man in his mid-sixties was referred because of severely painful hands. His problem, diagnosed as arthritis, had progressed over a four-year period. In addition to the pain, his hands had become increasingly weak. His doctor had sent him to the rehabilitation department of a nearby teaching hospital, where he had participated in several exercise programs. However, the exercises had not increased or maintained his strength. When I saw him, he could barely hold his set of keys. His grip was so weak he was unable to shake my hand.

When I examined him, I noted that the tissues of both hands and forearms were tight and contracted. His tissues responded rapidly, and at the end of the two-hour treatment he happily reported that he had very little pain. I asked if he could now shake my hand, and he did so with a firm grip. He was delighted by his increased strength and decreased pain.

Soft Tissue Manipulation Techniques

If your hands and arms are weak and painful, refer to "Carpal Tunnel Syndrome." Other areas likely to be weakened by soft tissue dysfunction are the hips and knees. Refer to those sections for treatment suggestions.

Musician's Pain

Musicians stress their bodies by placing them in uncomfortable positions for long hours of practice year after year. Gradually, imperceptively at first, many find their techniques compromised by the development of tight, contracted tissues. For some, their careers end because of incapacitating pain and dysfunction.

Musicians, who devote years of their lives to aesthetic study, receive the same kinds of treatment for their pain that doctors dispense to the rest of the population. The treatment doctors dole out to their musician patients includes: exercise, rest, pain medication, cortisone injections, stretching, surgery, heat, splinting, and psychiatric care. But these have no effect in normalizing the extensive soft tissue dysfunction that takes place in the bodies of musicians.

A few years ago, I attended a symposium titled "Performing Arts Medicine: Issues in Diagnosis and Management." Many prestigious doctors were mentioned as presenters, among whom was Dr. A. Doctor A has an international reputation as a specialist in musicians' problems. Also mentioned as a presenter was Dr. B, a physician with considerable experience in the care of musicians and performing artists.

On the first day of the symposium, I had the opportunity of introducing myself to Dr. B. I was interested in what he thought of my approach to treating soft tissue dysfunction I found in musicians. But Dr. B did not seem to be interested in my approach or what I had found. After a moment or two, he walked off, the usual reaction of doctors.

The last session of the symposium was interesting, however. That session was cochaired by Dr. A and Dr. B. After a few prefatory remarks, the session was thrown open to the audience. Immediately, a woman rose and tearfully related that she had been a woodwind soloist, but over a ten-year period she had developed severe and progressive pain and tightness in her upper back and both arms. Eventually the pain and tightness had become so severe that she had to give up her career as a musician. At this point, she broke down completely, and it took her a minute or two before she could compose herself.

She continued, telling the doctors and the rest of us that after her career as a soloist ended, she began to teach, but even that was becoming increasingly difficult because of excruciating pain. She had heard of the symposium and the doctors that would be there, and had attended to ask the doctors what they could do to help her.

Well, I thought, here it comes. Now I will learn what these eminent, top-of-the-line doctors do to treat musicians. I had my own thoughts as to how I would treat this woman—softening and normalizing the tight, contracted, fibrotic tissue that undoubtedly was the cause of her pain and dysfunction. Now I would learn what the doctors' approach would be.

I was astonished when Dr. A told this suffering musician that nothing could be done for her. Her case was much too advanced for anything to help her. If she had come to them a few years earlier, maybe something could have been done. Dr. B agreed.

The woman thanked them, murmuring that was what she thought they would say but had come down anyway just in case. She sat down, sobbing.

That was unfortunate because there was a great deal that could be done for this woman. I had successfully treated many people who had considerably worse symptoms than she described. Yet the doctors told this woman her case was hopeless.

I was in a dilemma. Should I stand and say I thought I could help her? Based on my extensive experience with doctors, as exemplified by the brief encounter with Dr. B at the coffee break, I decided against it. I didn't want to be disruptive. I determined instead to go over to her immediately after the session ended, give her my card, and tell her that I could offer her at least a glimmer of hope.

Next, a young man stood and stated he was a guitarist and that over the past two years was gradually developing pain and tightness in his arms and hands. He could still play well, but his technique was beginning to become affected. He asked the doctors for their help.

Now, I thought, I would learn the doctors' approach to treating a musician. Here was a musician presenting with early signs of pain and dysfunction. I leaned forward in my chair and eagerly awaited their remarks.

Dr. A told this musician the same thing he had told the previous one. His case was too advanced. If he had come earlier, maybe something could have been done, but now it was too late. Nothing could be done to help him. Dr. B agreed.

This was too much. The musician had early, *easily* treatable dysfunction. I could picture the condition of the tissues of his arms and hands and how they would respond to care. I couldn't believe the doctors had told him that nothing could be done. I determined to also talk with him after the session ended.

At the close of the session, I did go up to both musicians. I told them I could offer some help. I handed each a card and asked them to call me. Neither did.

Over the years, I have been puzzling over the response of the doctors to the entreaties of the two suffering musicians. How could the doctors not have suggested appropriate treatment? Then I realized the doctors didn't treat musicians; they managed them, just as the symposium said: "Performing Arts Medicine: Issues in Diagnosis and *Management*."

Case History 1

A young woman called one day. She had been a harpsichordist with a promising career, but two years earlier, while preparing for an important concert, her hands and arms became painfully tight, and she found that she was unable to play at all. She had been to several doctors, but nothing could be done for her. She had reluctantly come to the realization that she would never play again.

She had recently heard of me from a musician friend I had helped and called to see if I could help her also. She lived several hours away and could only come down on weekends. When she arrived for her first treatment, I learned that for several weeks before her final concert preparation she had been under a severe emotional strain because of a serious illness in her family. That, together with the additional emotional and physical stress of strenuous rehearsals, had put the finishing touches on a condition that had probably been developing over a long period of time.

When I examined her, I found that the tissues of her neck, back, shoulders, forearms, wrists, and fingers were tight, contracted, and painful to light palpation. The tissues of her hands and fingers were thick and painful, and she could only move her fingers slowly, with great pain.

I treated her for five weekends, in four- to five-hour sessions. At the end of this time, the affected tissues had softened appreciably and she could move her fingers with very little pain. She started to play again. She was delighted. I wanted to continue treating until her body was completely normalized, but she was pleased that she could play again. Since she no longer had aspirations of resuming a serious career, she was satisfied with her level of recovery, and treatments were discontinued.

Case History 2

A flutist who contacted me said that twenty years earlier she had injured the distal joint (the end joint) of her little finger. The joint had remained stiff over the years and in the past couple of years had stiffened even more. The area around the joint was becoming increasingly painful, and her technique was becoming affected.

She had heard of my work from another musician and wondered if I could help her. I found that there was fibrotic development around her affected joint, which prevented it from moving properly. The limited area of tissue dysfunction responded very rapidly to treatment, and she was completely pain- and symptom-free in three sessions and needed no further treatment.

Case History 3

A young woman, a pre-med student, was experiencing severe pain in her left (dominant) arm, such that it was seriously affecting her note-taking. She had heard of my work and was calling to make an appointment. I told her I would need a doctor's prescription in order to treat her. When she came for her first treatment, I learned that she had been a serious student of the violin; however, after several years of long hours of practice, her body and left arm had gradually become so painful that four years earlier she had to stop playing altogether.

Now that she was a pre-med student and had begun serious note-taking, the old pain had flared up with a vengeance. Even just a moment or two of note-taking caused excruciating, disabling pain. She was greatly concerned that the same pain that had ended her career as a violinist was now ending her opportunity of becoming a doctor.

When I examined her, I found contracted and painful tissue at her neck, left pectoral area, shoulder girdle, and down through her left arm and into her hand and fingers. Her pain rapidly reduced within two weeks, allowing her to do serious note-taking, but it took two months of treatment to normalize the severely contracted tissue of her pectoral, cervical, and shoulder girdle areas so she would have no problems in the future.

At the time of discharge, she was completely pain- and symptom-free. I do not know if she resumed her violin playing, but her dysfunctioning tissues had been normalized and she was fully capable of doing so.

Soft Tissue Manipulation Techniques

Your problem may be occurring anywhere in your body. Frequently, shoulders, arms, and hands are involved. Refer to "Carpal Tunnel Syndrome" for treatment suggestions. The neck, back, and hips are also likely areas of tissue dysfunction and pain. Refer to those sections for treatment techniques.

Neck Pain

Soft tissue dysfunction frequently underlies neck pain. The pain can be caused by tissues directly associated to the neck or tissues that lie far from it.

Case History

I received a call from a twenty-eight-year-old woman who said she had been suffering excruciating neck pain for two years. The pain was continuous, with not a moment of relief since it started. She had been treated by five practitioners: three medical doctors, a chiropractor, and a physical therapist. None had been able to help (nothing had shown up on her X-rays or other tests), and her neck pain continued unabated.

She had given up all hope and had resigned herself to a life of pain when someone told her of my work. She asked if I thought I could help her. I suggested she get a doctor's prescription that would allow me to examine and treat her, and we would then see what might be done.

When she came in for treatment, I learned she had been extremely busy with a computer project for three years. The only pain she was aware of was severe pain on the right side of her neck.

Her neck was so tender that at first she could not tolerate even the lightest touch there. When I applied lotion and gently examined the tissues of her right shoulder, arm, forearm, hand, and fingers, she was astonished at the severity of hidden pain that was revealed in those areas. She had not been aware of any pain before my gentle explorations.

Equally astonishing to her was the fact that when I touched those areas her neck pain became even more severe. There was also one small spot in the web of her thumb that seemed particularly connected to her neck pain. When I gently pressed it, her neck pain became unbearable. She was also surprised when I pointed out how tight and thick the muscles attached to her elbow were, as well as the tissues of her hand, fingers, and thumb. Dysfunctioning tissue was also found in her upper and mid-back, and down her left upper extremity, although not as severe as her right side.

After two hours of treatment, I noted that the tissues of her neck, back, and right upper extremity had softened, and she reported that her pain was almost gone and her body felt looser and lighter.

Her neck was so tender that at first she could not tolerate even the lightest touch there. When I applied lotion and gently examined the tissues of her right shoulder, arm, forearm, hand, and fingers, she was astonished at the severity of hidden pain that was revealed in those areas. There was also one small spot in the web of her thumb that seemed particularly connected to her neck pain.

She continued to respond rapidly and after only four more treatments was discharged, completely free of pain. I sent reports of her progress to her primary physician, the one who had sent her to those other practitioners, but did not receive a reply or query as to what I had done to successfully treat this previously "unhelpable" patient who had been prepared to live the rest of her life in excruciating pain.

Soft Tissue Manipulation Techniques

If your neck pain is caused by dysfunctioning soft tissue (organic or structural causation having been ruled out), then all areas that might be contributing to the pain must be examined and normalized.

Tissue areas most likely to cause neck pain include

1. the head
2. the neck itself
3. the upper back
4. the upper extremities.

For soft tissue manipulation techniques of the head, neck, and upper back refer to "Migraine and Muscle Contraction Headaches." For techniques that normalize the tissues of the upper extremities, refer to "Carpal Tunnel Syndrome."

Peripheral Vascular Disease

As a physical therapist, I have been involved with the care of ulcers (doctors and nurses refer to this as "wound care") caused by what doctors call peripheral vascular disease. My direct experience with this problem goes back almost half a century.

Not once in all these years have I seen a doctor carefully examine the tissues of a patient suffering from peripheral vascular disease. The reader may find it difficult to believe that not one doctor responded to my entreaty to even *touch* those tissues; nevertheless, this is so.

A question I have asked doctors repeatedly over the years is, "What is peripheral vascular disease?" There is usually some hesitation before an answer is given, which usually runs along the line of: "Peripheral vascular disease is a problem caused by fatty deposits that narrow blood vessels." I then ask, "How do you examine a patient suffering peripheral vascular disease?" The response is invariably the same: "I check the pressure at various levels of the limb."

"Peripheral vascular disease" as a diagnostic category is in fact a vague and imprecise term. I contend the problem primarily occurs when blood vessels are squeezed by tight, contracted tissues that *surround* them. Doctors are unaware of this because they do not carefully touch their patients.

As years pass and the tissues become increasingly tight and contracted, they exert an increasing tourniquet effect on the blood vessels that pass through them, making their job of supplying blood to the tissues of the extremity and of returning it to the heart increasingly difficult.

If the problem is arterial, the tissues from the calf down are tight and contracted. Arteries and their subdivisions are squeezed, and the limb, deprived of vital nutrients, becomes progressively desiccated and unhealthy. Ulcers form, and the life of the limb is put at great peril. Some arterial problems are indeed associated with fatty deposits, but I suspect that, even with these, contracted tissues surrounding the blood vessels are a contributing factor.

In the case of veins, as they become less able to do their job, the tissues that rely on them to remove fluid become congested and swollen. When doctors discuss venous problems, as in varicose veins, they say the valve leaflets fail. However, they don't understand that the primary cause of peripheral venous failure is dysfunctioning tissue outside the veins. When the tissues of the gluteal area and upper thigh become contracted and squeeze the veins, the venous return becomes difficult. Over time, the back-pressure of trying to return blood through the mass of tight and contracted tissues causes the valves to eventually fail.

The medical community's approach to arterial peripheral vascular disease is to dispense medication or attempt mechanical procedures designed to dilate the squeezed blood vessels. When these attempts fail, a surgical blood-vessel bypass may be needed, according to conventional doctors. This produces a painful, debilitating, and generally unspectacular outcome because the problem that caused the whole thing—tight, contracted, fibrotic tissue—has remained untreated. Venous peripheral vascular disease is currently dealt with—ineffectively—by applying constricting bandages or stockings to the bloated areas.

The effective treatment for tight, contracted, fibrotic tissues of an extremity is to soften and normalize the dysfunctioning tissues so the blood vessels can efficiently perform their job in a healthy environment. When this is done, the results can be surprisingly beneficial, even in advanced cases. The optimum time to soften and normalize tight tissues of the extremities is early on, before pain, swelling, and ulcers develop. However, proper treatment can be dramatically effective even in late stages.

It is unfortunate that patients suffering the health risk of so-called peripheral vascular disease are being subjected to costly, debilitating, ineffective, and painful surgeries (that include amputation) instead of being offered timely and effective treatment.

Case History

A woman in her eighties was referred for treatment. Her daughter had heard of my work and had arranged for the doctor's referral. She told me her mother suffered from peripheral vascular disease of forty years' duration. The pain had worsened as the years had gone by. Medications had not helped reduce the pain or prevent the progress of the problem.

Recently, the pain had become unbearable. She had difficulty taking even a few steps and was unable to get in or out of bed or chairs without help. She was living with her daughter, but because of her growing dysfunction, they were considering a nursing facility.

When I examined her legs, I could see that from mid-calf down to her feet, the skin was a brownish red. When I palpated this area, I found that the tissue was tough and leathery, and it almost had the feel of wood; there was no suppleness or softness of the skin and underlying tissue. I could see that, at the juncture where the skin became discolored and hardened, there was an indented line separating it from the tissues above. Farther up from the calves, from her knees to thighs, the tissues were tight and contracted, although not as hardened as the tissue in her calves. All of these areas were tender and painful to even the mildest touch.

I worked on her legs three times a week for two months. At first, she could tolerate only the mildest of treatments. But gradually the tissues softened, and there were indications that the circulation was improving. There was less pain, and the discoloration began to clear; the tissues became pink, at first for just a few seconds, then for a few minutes. Later, as treatment continued, dramatic improvement lasted for several hours between treatments.

By the second month of treatment, she felt improved enough to have the treatments discontinued. At that time, she was experiencing minimal pain, could get in and out of bed and chairs alone, and felt well enough to continue living with her daughter. She told me that she wished she had had this treatment forty years earlier. It was indeed sad that she hadn't.

Soft Tissue Manipulation Techniques

Before you treat yourself, I urge you to visit a doctor to rule out any underlying problem, such as phlebitis or deep vein thrombosis, that would preclude tissue manipulation. Always be alert to an area that is warm and red. If you notice this, stop treatment and check with your doctor.

Refer to sections titled "Hip Pain and Degenerative Joint Disease," "Knee Pain," and "Shin Splints" for soft tissue manipulation techniques. Be patient and gentle when you treat; don't rush.

Rotator Cuff Syndrome

The upper extremity moves through a wide range of motion. The shallow socket of the shoulder joint allows this free movement. The job of holding the upper extremity in place is assigned to muscles and ligaments closely associated with the shoulder joint. These comprise the rotator cuff.

When pain and physical dysfunction occur at the shoulder, doctors have developed the notion that the problem is a local one. They direct their surgeries, drugs, and painful stretches exclusively to this small area. Indeed, these tissues are subjected to trauma and wear and tear, and may well be the cause of shoulder dysfunction.

But it is just as likely that the underlying problem is extensive areas of tissue dysfunction well away from the shoulder. These distant tissues, as well as the rotators themselves, are likely to respond to soft tissue treatment. Therefore, before any surgical procedure is performed, soft tissue dysfunction should either be ruled out or properly treated. Otherwise, the doctor is risking surgical mutilation of the patient.

Case History 1

I received a call from a woman who said she was suffering from rotator cuff syndrome. She had fallen three months earlier. Doctors had diagnosed the resulting pain and difficulty in moving her shoulder as rotator cuff syndrome. They gave her pain medicine and other medications. In addition, they ordered physical therapy in the form of exercises and stretches; some of the shoulder stretches were applied by pulley. After each physical therapy session, the pain became more severe, and, as the pain worsened, her ability to move her arm became more difficult.

She said she was now unable to use her arm for any activity. When she attempted to move her shoulder, the pain became unbearable. Her doctors suggested surgery, but she was resigned to live with her pain rather than have an operation. A friend told her of my work, and she called to see if I could help. I told her I would need a doctor's prescription to examine and treat her. She said she would get one, and we arranged an appointment time.

When she arrived, I noted that she held her arm rigidly to her side. She felt constant pain, and the slightest movement caused the pain to increase. I found that the tissues of her neck, upper back, right chest, and the tissues of her entire right upper extremity from her shoulder down to her hand were spasmed.

Her tissues responded rapidly to treatment. As I worked down from her neck to shoulder to hand, I could feel the tissues softening under my fingers. After two hours, all the treated tissues felt soft and supple. She reported that "the pain had eased." When she sat up, I asked if she could now move her arm. To her astonishment, she moved her arm through a completely normal range of motion without any pain whatever.

I saw her two more times, but there was no return of pain or tissue spasm. She was discharged, delighted and happy. I reported her recovery to the doctor who had signed her prescription, but there was no response or inquiry as to what I had done to achieve that nonsurgical success.

Case History 2

A physical therapist contacted me with a complaint of pain and tightness of his right shoulder. He had been active years earlier in amateur softball and felt the stress of this activity was responsible for his shoulder problem, which had been diagnosed as rotator cuff syndrome. The modalities that had been prescribed had not helped, and his motivation and expertise in performing exercises and stretches had not prevented the pain and tightness from worsening, so he decided to try the surgery his doctor recommended. Unfortunately, the pain and tightness continued. That was three years ago.

He knew of my interest in soft tissue dysfunction and wondered if I might be able to help him. He had already obtained a doctor's prescription, so we scheduled a treatment session.

When he arrived for treatment, I noted that he had a thirty percent loss of shoulder movement. Examination revealed that the tissues surrounding his right scapula (shoulder blade) were severely contracted and fibrotic. The skin was adherent to the underlying tissues there. I noted the surgical scar, which was also adherent to underlying tissues.

In addition, I found the tissues of his neck, upper back, and down his right upper extremity were also severely contracted and fibrotic. The tissues of his left upper extremity were also contracted, but to a lesser degree.

His fibrotic tissues responded slowly to treatment; however, in three months, he was discharged, pain-free and with a full range of motion.

Case History 3

A woman called and said that her daughter, a high school student, was a swimmer but had injured her shoulder the previous season and now was unable to swim competitively. Her doctor had diagnosed the problem as rotator cuff syndrome. She had been given medication, including two cortisone injections, and had gone to a physical therapist for several sessions of exercise and stretches. However, despite these treatments, the pain had grown worse. Her daughter had not been able to complete the previous season and now was very upset because of the prospect of not being able to swim at all the current season, her final year of high school.

The woman knew of my work because I had helped a classmate of her daughter's, and she wondered if I might also be able to help her child. I told her to get a doctor's prescription, and we set up an appointment.

When I applied lotion and examined the tissues of the young swimmer, I did not find considerable soft tissue dysfunction. There was some spasm of the deltoid, the muscle at the top of the shoulder. But, interestingly, there was a small, hard knot about a quarter of an inch in diameter in the center of the muscle. I asked if she knew what that knot was. She said, "Oh, that must have been where they gave me an antibiotic injection a year ago." I asked to see how much shoulder movement she had, and she winced with pain when she attempted to raise her arm.

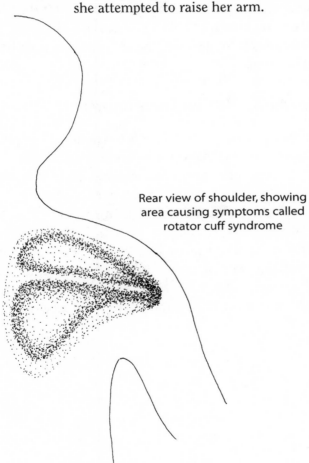

Rear view of shoulder, showing area causing symptoms called rotator cuff syndrome

I worked on her deltoid and its associated tissues for forty minutes and then asked if her arm was any better. She and her mother were surprised and delighted when she moved her arm through a complete range of motion without any pain whatever. Her mother asked if they could have some of that lotion, which she felt must have some sort of magical power to produce such an immediate and dramatic effect. I explained that it was ordinary lotion but gave her some anyway when I saw disbelief on her face.

When they returned for treatment two days later, her daughter was in tears because severe pain had returned. However, I noted the spasm had lessened and the knot was softer. At the end of the session, there was again full movement without pain. With each succeeding treatment, there was less return of pain and spasm. By the sixth session, there was no return of pain or spasm and the knot had disappeared. She was able to swim well the entire season, completely pain- and symptom-free.

Soft Tissue Manipulation Techniques

The same tissue areas responsible for symptoms of frozen shoulder are likely the areas that cause rotator cuff syndrome.

Treat the tissues of your upper extremity first. Refer to "Carpal Tunnel Syndrome" for soft tissue manipulation techniques.

Now treat your chest area. Refer to "Treating your chest" in the section titled "Migraine and Muscle Contraction Headaches."

Then treat your upper to lower back tissues. For soft tissue manipulation techniques of the upper back, refer to "Treating your neck and upper back" in the "Migraine and Muscle Contraction Headaches" section. For the lower back, refer to "Back Pain."

Scars

Scars, whether they have been caused by surgical incision, trauma, or burns, can "hold" pain for years and can be important components of physical dysfunction. Conventional doctors apparently are unaware of this.

Case History 1

A woman in her fifties was referred because of pain and extreme tightness of her neck and upper back. She said she had had this problem for as long as she could remember, and that it had worsened as time went on. Pain medication and muscle relaxants had not helped. Nor had ultrasound, heat, stretches, or exercises. The prescription I received from her doctor called for more of the same, but I called his office and was able to have the prescription changed to allow me to treat her properly.

Palpation revealed severely thickened and contracted tissues of her mid- and upper back, neck, and scalp. These tissues stubbornly resisted treatment, but gradually, after two months of deep work twice a week, her tissues softened, and she felt significant relief.

But not complete relief. We would get her tissues relaxed and softened after a treatment, but by the time she returned for her next treatment, much of the tightness had returned. I felt frustrated by this unusual retightening and began to explore other areas that might be triggering this response.

When I looked at her left cheek, just in front of her ear, I noticed that the skin was flat, whiter than the rest of her face, with the diameter of a quarter. I asked if she knew what that whitish area was. She said that when she was three, she had fallen against a hot cookstove, and the whitish area was what remained of the burn scar.

I gently touched and palpated the scar tissue. At first, there was no sensation. But in a moment or two, she began to experience intense, excruciating pain. At the same time, she began to feel strong sensations radiating down into her neck and left arm.

Gradually the pain in the scar tissue and the sensations down her neck eased. As I worked on the scar tissue, it came into her mind that her left neck and arm had "always been weak" since childhood.

At the next session, she reported that there had been only a slight return of tightness in her neck and back. After a few more sessions, she was discharged, pain- and symptom-free.

I was astonished that a scar that had occurred fifty years earlier could hold so much pain and cause significant physical dysfunction. It certainly demonstrated the importance of examining and treating scar tissue.

Case History 2

A woman called and said it was becoming increasingly difficult for her to swallow. Food and medicine stuck in her throat. The problem had become increasingly severe over the past several months. Doctors thought her problem was caused by panic attacks, but she felt she panicked when she couldn't swallow. She heard of my work and asked if I could help her. I told her to get a doctor's prescription, and we set up an appointment.

I carefully checked the tissues of her throat and detected a small, hard, indurated area on the left side. It felt like a scar. I asked her about it, and she said that several years earlier her neck had been cut by some falling glass. When I pressed on the scar, she felt sensations radiating into her throat. The scar responded rapidly to care and in two weeks had completely softened. By the end of this treatment period, she could swallow normally without any difficulty.

Case History 3

I was treating a woman for an upper extremity problem. During one session, I discovered a bit of hard tissue about the diameter of a quarter at the front of her chest just below her collarbone. As I gently palpated this area, she began to cough violently. She told me she was a real estate agent and was frequently embarrassed when she was with clients by paroxysms of severe coughing that lasted for several minutes. This had been going on for years, but she had not been aware of this cough-triggering bit of tissue.

Every time I pressed on it, she began to cough. For the next several sessions, I worked to normalize this scarlike tissue. As it gradually softened, the violence of her reactive coughing lessened. Finally, the coughing completely ceased. At the last session, the cause of her problem suddenly came into her mind. She recalled that when she was three she had had a severe case of whooping cough. She remembered the bouts of violent coughing and how it made her chest hurt.

I carefully checked the tissues of her throat and detected a small, hard, indurated area on the left side. It felt like a scar. The scar responded rapidly to care and in two weeks had completely softened. By the end of this treatment period, she could swallow normally without any difficulty.

Apparently, the trauma of coughing had injured her tissues and caused a scar to form. The scar had then retriggered the coughing episodes when the stress of dealing with clients caused the tissues surrounding the scar to tighten.

She called a few months later to let me know that she no longer experienced the embarrassing coughing episodes.

These three cases demonstrate the importance of reducing all scar tissue early on so future complications can be avoided.

Soft Tissue Manipulation Techniques

Scar tissue can trigger pain and physical dysfunction. All scar tissue, whether caused by burns, trauma, or surgical incisions, should be treated and released, thereby avoiding this possibility. Soft tissue manipulation techniques such as rippling, circles, back-and-forths, kneading, and nudges are effective; refer to the glossary for instructions.

Start your treatment sessions with extreme gentleness, as there may be considerable hidden pain locked up in the scar. Work slowly, be patient, and allow plenty of time. If the scar is thick and extensive, be prepared to treat in extended sessions for several weeks or months.

Sciatica

When the tissues of the gluteal area become tight and contracted, the pain receptors there are squeezed, causing the sensation of pain. The sciatic nerve passes through the region; therefore, doctors call pain in that area sciatica. However, tissue dysfunction rarely occurs in just one small area of the body.

Case History

A man in his late thirties was referred for treatment of severe sciatica. When I chatted with him before treatment, I learned that his painful sciatica had been developing over the past several months but that he had another problem that had been plaguing him for four years.

He told me he formerly enjoyed participating in martial arts but four years earlier had torn his tensor fascia lata when doing a karate kick. This injury forced him to stop his martial arts activity.

The tensor fascia lata is a thick, tough band of connective tissue that runs from the hip down to the knee. It is frequently involved in hip and knee problems but is so tough I could not imagine a karate kick could tear it. I asked him how he knew it was torn. He said that, at the time, he was living in Boston and, as he wanted to have the very best care for his athletic injury, he went to the physician treating a particular athletic organization of great renown. The doctor diagnosed his problem as a "torn tensor fascia lata."

The doctor prescribed a course of treatment consisting of ultrasound, heat, massage, exercise, and stretching. This regimen was diligently pursued for six months, but the pain and other symptoms worsened to such an extent that treatment was eventually discontinued. Nothing else was offered, so my patient continued to live in severe pain during the intervening years.

When I examined him, I found that the tissues of his gluteal area, particularly on the right side, down his right thigh and into his right knee, were contracted and painful to light touch. The tissues adjacent to his tensor fascia lata were particularly painful.

I asked him if his current doctor thought there might be some relationship between his "torn" tensor fascia lata and his painful sciatica. He told me he had wondered that himself, but his doctor said no, they were two distinctly separate issues.

I treated him intensively three times a week for two weeks. At the end of that time, he no longer had sciatic pain, and the symptoms relating to his tensor fascia lata had diminished.

He told me he was interested in getting every iota of his tensor fascia lata problem eliminated until there was not the slightest "twinge" of a problem. So we continued treatment, at decreasing frequency, for a total of three months. At the end of this time, he did not have the slightest twinge, and I discharged him from treatment, completely pain- and symptom-free, pleased and happy.

I called him two years following discharge, and he reported that there had been no return of either sciatica or tensor fascia lata pain. He had not returned to martial arts but felt he was physically able to do so.

Here is an example of a doctor in charge of athletes, displaying the same ignorance of soft tissue dysfunction that doctors in charge of the general population display. If my patient had been a professional athlete, dancer, or other specialized performer, his career would have been ruined. Think of all the unfortunate individuals whose careers have been ruined.

Soft Tissue Manipulation Techniques

Refer to "Back Pain" for appropriate treatment techniques. For treatment of the tensor fascia lata, refer to "Knee Pain."

Shin Splints

The job assigned to the muscle group located at the shin is to lift the foot at each step. Unfortunately, this muscle, the anterior tibialis, is a small one and is easily overworked by the strenuous process of running. Over time, this muscle and its associated tissues becomes contracted, thickened, and painful. Doctors refer to this condition as shin splints. However, as with most soft tissue problems, other tissue areas become involved. Indeed, by the time an individual experiences pain and dysfunction of the shin tissues, the entire lower extremity has become dysfunctional.

Doctors, however, attempt to treat shin splints with rest, drugs, and, believe it or not, surgery! Directing attention and treatment exclusively to the area of the shin is to render a gross disservice to the athlete. To mutilate those dysfunctioning tissues with a sharp scalpel demonstrates a high level of ignorance. Proper treatment is to soften and normalize all dysfunctioning tissue so pain will go away and the body can become healthy once again.

Case History

I received a call from someone who said he was a serious runner. He had been unable to run for the past two weeks because of severe shin splints. The problem had plagued him for some time but had worsened over the past three months. He had been to a few doctors, but they had been unable to help him.

His immediate concern was a ten-mile run that was coming up in a week. He had his heart set on participating in the event, but, because of his painful shins, he feared he would not be able to run. Someone had mentioned my work, and he was calling to ask if I could help. I told him to get a doctor's prescription that would enable me to examine and treat, then we set up an appointment for the following day.

When I examined him, I found that all the tissues of both his lower extremities were tight and contracted, particularly so from his knees down through his ankles and into his feet. The tissues of both calves were extremely tight and painful to mild palpation. But most dysfunctioning of all was the condition of the tissues of his shins, which were almost as hard as wood. The skin was tightly adherent to underlying tissues. When I applied lotion, I could feel thick, well-defined, fibrotic bands throughout. The lightest palpation caused excruciating pain.

I felt I could help him with a series of treatments, but was uncertain if we should start so soon before his important event. My treatment, by softening and normalizing his contracted tissues, could possibly bring to the surface considerable amounts of hidden pain that his body had accommodated itself to, which would make the ten-mile run, now only five days off, even more difficult to tolerate. On the other hand, the softened and normalized tissues might become completely pain-free and he could run without difficulty. It is difficult to predict tissue response of the first few treatments.

After discussing the matter with me, he decided to go ahead with a treatment, because he certainly was unable to run in his present condition. The tissues of his thighs and calves softened considerably. The tissues of his shins, however, were more resistant, and did not soften to the same extent. At the end of the treatment, he said that his legs were free of pain and were "feeling pretty good." That was on Monday.

He called on Wednesday to give me a status report. His legs were completely pain-free the evening of the treatment, but on Tuesday

Extensive areas of tissue dysfunction underlie what is called "shin splints."

morning he experienced moderate pain in both shins. This pain eased as the day went on. When he awoke on Wednesday morning, his legs were free of pain and he thought he would try a five-mile run. He finished his five miles without any pain or discomfort, but afterwards began to feel some pain creeping back.

Again, there was the dilemma of whether or not to give another treatment before the ten-mile run on Saturday. I felt that it might be best to hold off until after the run. He was feeling pretty good and I didn't want to take a chance of releasing more hidden pain.

He called on Monday to say that the ten-mile run went well, and that he had no pain or discomfort. I was greatly relieved to hear this. After this, I treated him for one month. The tissues of his shins and calves softened appreciably, and we extended treatment up to his hips. When discharged, he was running well with no complaints. I told him to call if he had any recurrence of symptoms. That was several months ago. No call yet.

Soft Tissue Manipulation Techniques

Soft tissue dysfunction that underlies what is called shin

splints can extend from the hips (or even higher) down into the ankle and foot. Those dysfunctioning tissues are also causative of knee pain. For soft tissue manipulation suggestions, refer to "Knee Pain."

Sinus Headache

Although many patients refer to their pain as "sinus headaches," their doctors deny the occurrence of sinus-generated headaches. In my experience, it is the patients who are correct. When a patient complains of sinus headache, I first check the "sinus areas" adjacent to both sides of the nose (see "Sinus Pain"). I move out from these to investigate other areas for tight, fibrotic tissue. These are usually found on the face, frequently at the temporal and forehead areas, although the scalp, neck and upper back may also be involved. When all of these are reduced and normalized, the sinus headaches go away.

Case History

A woman in her late fifties came to me because of excruciating sinus pain she had endured for several years. She also suffered from what her doctors diagnosed as severe migraine headaches. The two problems were thought by her doctors to be separate. Over the years, she had been given various medicines and painkillers, all to no avail. The sinus pain and headaches grew worse and worse.

Finally, extensive surgery on her sinus cavities was performed. Sadly, this surgery also had no effect on her excruciating sinus pain and headaches, which continued unabated. Someone told her of my work, and she obtained the necessary doctor's referral.

When she reported for treatment, she stated that she was experiencing severe sinus pain and a severe headache. My examination revealed that the tissues overlying the front of her left face and cheek were hard, indurated, and extremely painful to the touch. I found contracted, fibrotic tissue extending from her sinus area to her left temple and up into her scalp. She reported that when I palpated these tissues her headache immediately worsened. She stated that none of the doctors, over the several years they had treated her, had ever examined or touched any of them.

I worked on the tight, contracted tissues, and as I did so, she reported that her sinus and headache pain was decreasing. By the end of the first treatment, she no longer had any pain whatsoever. She felt this was a miracle. I gave her two more treatments and discharged her, pain-free and very happy. I checked with her two years later, and she reported that she remained free of any pain.

Soft Tissue Manipulation Techniques

Lie on your back with your upper body comfortably propped up by pillows or a bolster. Have lotion

Dysfunctioning areas that cause sinus headache pain

187

and a cup of warm water standing by. Apply a small amount of lotion to each wedge and explore. Begin your exploration using your forefingers as probes. Use circles, back-and-forths, and nudges as described in the glossary.

Is one side thicker? Is one or both hard and stiff? Do you find small, hard knots? These are bits of fibrotic tissue that will soften as treatment proceeds.

Place a finger next to your nose and run your thumb across the skin of a wedge. Is the skin thick? Does the skin ripple as your thumb is drawn toward your finger, or is it bound down to underlying tissue? Try the other wedge. Is the skin thicker? Less thick? More adherent to underlying tissues? Less adherent?

Grasp a wedge between thumb and forefinger. Can you move it about, or is it too thick and stiff? Can you nudge it with your forefinger? Try slow nudges, fast nudges. How about the other side—any difference?

If the lotion is drying out and getting sticky, add a bit more, or a drop or two of water, to get it slippery again. Perhaps you like the extra friction that you have with the drying lotion; it helps grip the skin when you maneuver it. If so, don't add lotion or water; use the friction to your advantage.

Explore each wedge thoroughly, from nose to cheekbone, and up and down—from the outer corner of your eye to the bottom of your cheekbone. Take your time; don't rush. When you have gained a sense of the tissues of your sinus areas, begin the treatment.

Reapply lotion, place your thumb under your jawbone for leverage, and sweep your finger slowly across the first wedge to be treated, down from the bone under your eye. Continue these sweeps until the entire wedge is covered. Take your time; don't rush. Repeat the movement several times. Keep your thumb where it is and use your finger to perform small circles over the wedge. Gradually enlarge the circles until each circle covers the entire wedge. Perform this movement several times. Is the wedge of tissue beginning to soften, to feel lighter? Now treat the wedge with small nudging movements.

Run your finger horizontally along the bone under your eye, from nose to cheekbone. Do you feel very small, hard, fibrotic knots in the skin and underlying tissues? These not only cause "bags" to form under your eyes but are also components of sinus problems. Treat these knots with small circles and up-and-downs. These tissue dysfunctions are stubborn and will require additional treatments before they soften and normalize.

After treating one sinus wedge, move over and treat the other one. After both wedges have been treated, finish with a gentle "towel rub."

After doing the techniques for normalization of the sinus areas, then explore and treat other areas of your face and head. You might also have to investigate your neck, upper back, and chest. If this is necessary, review the soft tissue manipulation techniques under "Migraine and Muscle Contraction Headaches."

Sinus Pain

Several years ago, I was treating a young man for an upper extremity problem. One day, he came to my office complaining of excruciating sinus pain. The pain was so severe he was in tears. The only thing I could think to do was to have him lie down and to gently place my hands on his face where he was hurting. This seemed to give him some relief, so I was encouraged to move my fingers in small circles on both sides of his face adjacent to his nose, the areas of his pain. To my surprise and his delight, he reported that his pain was receding and he could feel that his sinuses were draining. Since that time, I have successfully treated numbers of patients who complained of sinus pain.

Case History

I was once the owner of a large rehabilitation group in Southern California and needed to hire a physical therapist for a particular treatment center. I knew of an excellent therapist and took him to lunch. When I discussed the position, he said he was fairly satisfied with his present job. Besides, he informed me that he was at the moment experiencing excruciating sinus pain and was finding it difficult to concentrate. He told me that he had suffered severe sinus pain for several years and nothing had helped the problem. I asked, if I were able to effectively treat his sinus pain, would he come to work for me? He answered with an emphatic yes!

We stopped by my office, and I proceeded to treat his sinuses (after he had called his doctor to get the permission necessary for me to treat him). As I did, I gathered from his demeanor that he was skeptical of what I was doing. At the end of forty minutes, he reported that there was no change in the amount of pain he was experiencing, and he left the office. I was extremely embarrassed by the lack of results.

However, later that afternoon he called and said that I had myself a therapist. Two hours after the treatment, he felt his sinuses open and drain. He said, "I don't know what you did, but it sure worked."

I gave him six more treatments. His sinus tissues were then soft, supple, and symptom-free. He readily learned to treat his own sinuses when retightening began, so there was no recurrence of pain or any other symptom in the three years he worked for me.

Soft Tissue Manipulation Techniques

The triangular-shaped wedges of tissue that lie on either side of the nose are what I call the "sinus areas." When lotion is applied to these areas,

Dysfunctioning areas that cause sinus pain

191

thick, fibrotic skin and underlying tissue is invariably revealed. When these thickened tissues are softened and normalized, symptoms of pain and congestion recede and disappear.

Lie on your back with your upper body comfortably propped up by pillows or a bolster. Have lotion and a cup of warm water standing by. Apply a small amount of lotion to each wedge and explore. Begin your exploration using your forefingers as probes. Use circles, back-and-forths, and nudges as described in the glossary.

Is one side thicker? Is one or both hard and stiff? Do you find small, hard knots? These are bits of fibrotic tissue that will soften as treatment proceeds.

Place a finger next to your nose and run your thumb across the skin of a wedge. Is the skin thick? Does the skin ripple as your thumb is drawn toward your finger, or is it bound down to underlying tissue? Try the other wedge. Is the skin thicker? Less thick? More adherent to underlying tissues? Less adherent?

Grasp a wedge between thumb and forefinger. Can you move it about, or is it too thick and stiff? Can you nudge it with your forefinger? Try slow nudges, fast nudges. How about the other side— any difference?

If the lotion is drying out and getting sticky, add a bit more, or a drop or two of water, to get it slippery again. Perhaps you like the extra friction that you have with the drying lotion; it helps grip the skin when you maneuver it. If so, don't add lotion or water; use the friction to your advantage.

Explore each wedge thoroughly, from nose to cheekbone, and up and down—from the outer corner of your eye to the bottom of your cheekbone. Take your time; don't rush. When you have gained a sense of the tissues of your sinus areas, begin the treatment.

Reapply lotion, place your thumb under your jawbone for leverage, and sweep your finger slowly across the first wedge to be treated, down from the bone under your eye. Continue these sweeps until the entire wedge is covered. Take your time; don't rush. Repeat the movement several times. Keep your thumb where it is and use your finger to perform small circles over the wedge. Gradually enlarge the circles until each circle covers the entire wedge. Perform this movement several times. Is the wedge of tissue beginning to soften, to feel lighter? Now treat the wedge with small nudging movements.

Run your finger horizontally along the bone under your eye, from nose to cheekbone. Do you feel very small, hard, fibrotic knots in the skin and underlying tissues? These not only cause "bags" to form under your eyes but are also components of sinus problems. Treat these knots with small circles and up-and-downs. These tissue dysfunctions are stubborn and will require additional treatments before they soften and normalize.

After treating one sinus wedge, move over and treat the other one. After both wedges have been treated, finish with a gentle "towel rub."

Response to treatment varies widely. There can be immediate and dramatic relief, such as severe pain reduced to zero in a matter of minutes. At other times, pain relief is felt thirty minutes, or perhaps two or more hours, following treatment. I have had patients, treated in the morning, call late in the afternoon to tell me that their sinuses had just "opened" and were draining, with significant relief of pain. Some cases were more stubborn and required several visits. As with all soft tissue dysfunction, it is best to continue treatments until the tissues are soft and normalized, so symptoms are not likely to return.

Sprained Ankle

It is important to keep an open mind about any treatment model. Once practitioners get locked into a certain concept, they find it exceedingly difficult to let go of it. Take, for example, the treatment of sprained ankles.

Case History

At the end of her second week of treatment, a woman I was treating for an upper extremity problem came in one morning, limping painfully.

"Oh, no," I said. "What's happened now?"

She said her arm was fine but she had slipped the night before and sprained her ankle. She had just been to her doctor, who had examined her and wrapped her ankle in an Ace bandage. She hoped I could help and, knowing the system, had obtained a prescription from her doctor.

I said there was nothing I could do for a sprained ankle. I then recited the conventional wisdom about the treatment of a sprained ankle: "cold, then heat, plenty of rest, elevation, gradual weight bearing as tolerated." She persisted, however, in her request that I do something, or, at least, try to do something for her ankle. Finally, I relented.

I unwrapped and examined her ankle. It was swollen and painful for her to move. But to my surprise, when I palpated the tissues well above the ankle on up into her calf and then down into her heel and instep, I found the tissues in these areas to be spasmed and painful to light touch. I thought, "Why not try to soften these spasmed and painful areas?" So I proceeded to gently work on them. They responded quickly and in a few minutes began to relax and soften.

After thirty minutes, I asked her to get up and see how her ankle felt. To her delight and to my surprise, she no longer had any pain or discomfort. She thanked me and walked out without a limp. Since then, I have treated four other sprained-ankle patients with similar results.

What do these experiences point toward? Contrary to the commonly held assumption that it is the tendon at the ankle that is sprained when a sprained ankle occurs, I contend it is the soft tissues (muscle and fascia) attached to the ends of the tendon that are injured. When these fragile tissues are traumatized, they spasm. The spasm squeezes nerves and vascular structures, which in turn produces the pain and swelling. Tendons are strong and tough, not easily injured or susceptible to being sprained, whereas soft tissues by their very nature are susceptible to injury.

> *Contrary to the commonly held assumption that it is the tendon at the ankle that is sprained when a sprained ankle occurs, I contend it is the soft tissues (muscle and fascia) attached to the ends of the tendon that are injured. When these fragile tissues are traumatized, they spasm.*

Soft Tissue Manipulation Techniques

It never hurts to try, if you try in a gentle manner. My experience with treating sprained ankles has been limited but interesting. I see no harm in having others try similar gentle techniques. I urge you to have your injury checked to rule out the possibility of a fracture or some other severe injury before you start self-treatment.

Let's assume that your right ankle is affected. Lie on your left side with your upper body propped up on pillows or a bolster. This is so you can reach your ankle easily. Place some towels under the leg you are going to treat. Bend your knee and position your leg so it is as comfortable as possible. Apply some lotion to your calf up by your knee. Dilute it with a few drops of water so your treating hand can move gently and smoothly, without any friction, over the surface of your skin. Lubricate your entire leg from knee to toes in a similar manner.

Make gentle floats starting from about three inches above your ankle on up to your knee. Do this so gently that it causes no additional pain. If you feel increased pain, you probably are not doing it gently enough. Continue with these floats so all tissue surface is covered. Reposition your leg as necessary. If at any time you feel increased pain from what you are doing, back off and float with an even lighter touch. If even your lightest touch causes increased pain, then discontinue treatment. However, if you find that your tissues are relaxing and the pain is easing, then continue with the floats. With continued tissue relaxation, gently increase the intensity of treatment.

Now place your palm and fingers gently on your calf up by your knee, and, keeping them on that same spot, make gentle circles so that the deeper tissues there are gently moved. How did that feel? If it caused pain, then move even slower, with even more gentleness. If things are going well, move to another spot and do the same.

Continue until all tissues from knee to above the ankle have been moved in this gentle manner. If all is going well, then place your hands on opposite sides of the calf and make small circles in unison so that the tissues deep inside the calf are gently moved. Picture in your mind that you are gently moving your deeper calf tissues around your shinbone. Do you think your tissues are loosening? If so, increase the arc of the circles.

Now move down to the ankle itself. Gently place your palm on the outside anklebone. Don't do any moving; just place it there. How does it feel? If it doesn't hurt, make tiny, gentle circles with your palms. No pain? Then continue; if it hurts, discontinue. Now try the inside anklebone. If it feels okay, continue; if it hurts, discontinue.

Move down to your foot. Perform the same palmings. Continue until all areas of your foot have been gently treated. To finish, go back up to your knee and work down with circles. How do things feel now? They should feel better, and you should be more relaxed and feel less pain. Remember, at the slightest increase in pain, discontinue.

Tendinitis

Doctors blame tendons for all sorts of body pain. However, tendons are rarely a problem. The medical misdiagnosis of tendinitis is invariably bestowed upon individuals that suffer soft tissue dysfunction well away from the tendons and their protective sheaths. If doctors began carefully touching the bodies of their patients, they would understand this; as things stand, doctors attempt to treat misdiagnosed tendinitis with drugs and surgery.

Case History

The manager of a fast-food restaurant was referred for treatment. He brought in a prescription bearing the diagnosis "tendinitis, both heels." The young man told me he experienced severe, excruciating pain with each step. He had a bandage wound around each ankle to limit motion there. His shoes were loosely laced because of dreadful pain in both feet, and he walked slowly as if in severe pain.

I examined his legs and feet and found that the tissues of both legs from calf down through forefoot and into his toes were tight, contracted, fibrotic, and severely painful to the lightest palpation. Here was another case of extensive soft tissue dysfunction.

I told him I could feel contracted tissues and fibrotic fibers in his calves and feet and that there was a good possibility I might be able to help him by softening, releasing, and normalizing the dysfunctioning tissues. He said to go ahead with the treatment program I outlined.

I treated him for two weeks, three times a week. By this time, the affected tissues were normalized, and he was free of all pain. He walked quickly with no discomfort. When I discharged him at the end of the six sessions, he told me that at the first treatment, when I spoke of fibrotic fibers, he thought I was crazy because the whole thing sounded wacky. But now he had to admit that what I did had worked. Once again, tendons were blamed for what was really an extensive soft tissue problem.

Soft Tissue Manipulation Techniques

Doctors may mistakenly blame tendons for pain occurring anywhere in the body. Shoulders, elbows, hands, and heels are frequently misdiagnosed as having tendinitis. Refer to "Carpal Tunnel Syndrome" and "Shin Splints" for treatment suggestions. If you have been diagnosed as having tendinitis in another area of your body, refer to the appropriate section for treatment suggestions.

Tennis Elbow

Soft tissue dysfunction underlies complaints of body or headache pain and dysfunction, and usually the dysfunction is extensive in nature. This is true for what doctors call tennis elbow. Pain noted at the elbow is merely the tip of an extensive iceberg of soft tissue dysfunction. Tight and contracted tissues of the entire upper extremity and throughout large areas of the body are likely involved. When the dysfunctioning tissues are properly treated, the pain perceived at the elbow will go away.

Case History

A fifty-eight-year-old woman was referred for treatment. Her doctor had diagnosed her condition as tennis elbow. When I examined her, I found that the tissues of both upper extremities, neck, head, scalp, upper back, lower back, gluteal areas, and both lower extremities from her hips down to her toes were thick, tight, contracted, and severely painful. The tissues of her back were so thickened that I could not palpate her spinal column. Her shoulders were pulled painfully forward by contracted chest tissues.

She suffered from ear pain and tinnitus. Her body was so painful that she could do mild yard work for only fifteen minutes before dreadful pain shot up her legs into her back. She could sleep for only two to three hours at a time before the pain throughout her body awakened her. Her legs demonstrated significant development of peripheral vascular disease. She suffered from painfully severe bunions, and the tissues of both her hands were tight, thick, and painful. Yet, notwithstanding the fact that her entire body was severely painful, her doctor had diagnosed her problem simply as "tennis elbow."

I worked on her for eight months. When she was discharged, all her symptoms were significantly reduced. She could sleep for four to five hours and work in her garden for two to three hours before needing a rest. Her ear pain and tinnitus was reduced, as was much of the pain in the rest of her body, including her formerly painful elbow. I was so busy treating her many problem areas that I did not have time to deal with her peripheral vascular condition.

Eventually, however, she had surgery performed on her bunions. Her tissue dysfunction had progressed over the entirety of her life. When I saw her, it had become so severe that I could only more or less "patch things up," although she was pleased with the results of the treatments.

Soft Tissue Manipulation Techniques

The diagnosis of tennis elbow is a frivolous one, as demonstrated by the above case history. You will have to examine your body to find your dysfunctioning tissues. The tissues of your entire upper extremity are probably affected, so carefully check and treat from shoulder to fingers as described in "Carpal Tunnel Syndrome." The tissues of your neck and back are also likely areas. Refer to those sections for soft tissue manipulation suggestions.

Tinnitus

Tinnitus can be caused by a multitude of underlying problems that respond to medical treatment. However, after all medically understood problems have been ruled out, a large number of patients continue to experience severe symptoms and are told that "nothing more can be done." The continued suffering of these individuals may be caused by soft tissue dysfunction.

When I treat someone for neck and back problems, I frequently find that they also complain of tinnitus (a sensation of "ringing" in the ears), a feeling of stuffiness in the ears, and ear pain. Usually, the tinnitus is more severe in one ear. Investigation invariably reveals thickened, fibrotic tissue adjacent to the ear at the area of the attachment of the sternomastoid muscle, the long muscle that runs from the sternum (the breastbone) to just behind the ear. As a matter of fact, the substance of this muscle itself is frequently thick, tough, and hardened, especially where it attaches close to the ear.

A component of the neck and back treatment is directed toward the sternomastoid and the area of its attachment close to the ear. I find that as this tissue softens, patients state that ear symptoms, including tinnitus, diminish significantly. At times, they report that they no longer have any tinnitus, although this improvement to date has only been temporary. I have not been able to treat tinnitus for extended periods, because when the neck and back problems are successfully reversed, the patient is discharged; the reduction of tinnitus is a secondary benefit of treatment. I do not know for certain that tinnitus can be completely eliminated over a longer course of treatment specifically directed toward it, but I am confident that this could happen.

Case History

I treated a patient who suffered for years with loud ringing and uncomfortable pressure in her right ear.

When I first started treating the severe pain and tightness of her upper back and neck, her symptoms of tinnitus and pressure were "unbearable" and "terribly disruptive," as she put it. As treatment continued, at first twice a week and then every two to three weeks, she no longer had any symptom of pressure, and described her symptom of tinnitus as "usually mild," with occasional episodes at moderate levels. At times, she was completely unaware of any ringing.

As the excruciating body pain she experienced at the start of her care diminished and she came in for treatment less frequently, we spent just a few minutes of her two-hour treatment on her "tinnitus area." The improvement of her tinnitus problem slowed, as had the urgency to treat the problem. She was discharged from treatment when her back and neck pain was completely resolved, although she still experienced the reduced level of tinnitus.

Soft Tissue Manipulation Techniques

The primary area of soft tissue dysfunction that underlies tinnitus is the same as for ear pain, namely, the sternomastoid muscle. The tissues of the scalp, face, and upper back may also be involved. The treatment techniques are the same as for ear pain. It is likely that the fibrotic development at the attachment of the sternomastoid, just behind the ear, will be very thick, and will require extended treatment.

Lie on your back with your head comfortably supported by pillows. Arrange them so your head is tilted forward; this will produce some slack in your sternomastoids. Let us assume that your left ear is the painful one. You will turn your head to the left; this will further relax the muscle where it attaches behind your left ear.

Slip your right hand under your head so the palm of your hand supports the weight of your head. This will free your fingers and thumb to explore and treat. Start your treatment at the area of attachment with your first and second fingers held closely together, i.e., doubled. This makes them into a very effective probing instrument. Use them to perform circles and back-and-forths. Take your time; don't rush. Treat the entire area that surrounds your ear, paying particular attention to the tissue behind and below.

Are you finding thick tissue that becomes painful with gentle treatment? Move up into the scalp region. Let your fingers follow any pain or contracted areas. As you move outward, add multiple-finger movements.

Go back to the attachment and examine the sternomastoid itself. Move down and pincer it gently between thumb and bent forefinger as you go. Roll it gently, feeling for contracted, fibrotic or painful areas. Try some gentle single-finger circles, back-and-forths, and single-finger stationary presses. Move down to where the muscle attaches to the chest wall and examine and treat. Use single-finger, double-finger, and multiple-finger circles.

Explore and treat the tissues of your face. Let your fingers look for tight, contracted areas and for areas that cause any increase of your ear pain. Refer to "Ear Pain" for detailed instruction. For treatment of the upper back, refer to "Migraine and Muscle Contraction Headaches."

TMJ Pain

Tight, contracted tissues outside a joint can radiate pain perceived to be coming from inside the joint. Doctors apparently do not understand this and are therefore confused about the etiology of the pain they misnamed temporomandibular joint (TMJ) pain. Doctors attempt to treat TMJ pain and dysfunction with drugs, surgery, and crude stretching.

The jaw swings loosely from the skull, allowing wide opening and side-to-side movement, necessary for chewing food. The joint that allows this free movement is the temporomandibular joint; it's held in place by muscles attached to it, but these muscles and associated tissues may become tight, contracted, and fibrotic. The mouth cannot open fully, and pain is generated. As frequently happens with other joints, pain caused by soft tissues outside the joint is perceived to be coming from within the joint. Proper treatment is to normalize the tight, contracted tissues. When this is done, the mouth opens fully and the pain goes away.

Case History

When I first came to Charlottesville, Virginia, I heard of a plastic surgeon who was interested in finding a physical therapist who had experience in working with TMJ patients. I immediately phoned and told him I had such experience and was interested in treating patients with TMJ. I briefly outlined my nonsurgical approach that led to successful treatment of many patients that suffered jaw pain. I told him I would be pleased to stop by his office and discuss my treatment in greater detail.

He said he would not have time for such a conversation but would have his secretary take my name and phone number and would call me if the need ever arose.

Three years later, I received a call from a dentist who wanted to refer a patient suffering from severe TMJ who had been unresponsive to prior care. I asked how he had heard of me, and he said the plastic surgeon I had spoken to three years earlier had given him my name and phone number.

I told the dentist I would be pleased to treat his patient and that I was currently working with a modality called "microcurrent." I had used this electronic device for several months, had good results with it for a variety of problems, and it seemed promising in treating TMJ.

I told him my plan was to try the microcurrent intensively for two weeks. If it was not effective with this patient, then I would use techniques that I had found to be effective in the past. He said the plan was sound and that the patient already had a prescription allowing me to treat, and that I could start any time.

I immediately set up an appointment with the patient, an eighteen-year-old woman. I learned that she had been suffering a severely painful jaw for two years. She could open her mouth about one inch, barely enough to eat small bits of soft food slowly, and even minimal opening caused an increase in pain.

In addition, she suffered from a severe and continuous headache that had lasted two years already. Her headache was rated as ten on a scale of one to ten, and had started at the same time as her TMJ symptoms. Both problems progressed rapidly shortly after a severe emotional experience.

The plastic surgeon had performed two surgeries on her temporomandibular joints. The first one was an exploratory arthroscopic surgery, which was unsuccessful in providing any improvement of her problem.

Since her jaw pain and limited motion, and her severe head-ache, continued unabated, a second surgery was performed. This was an extensive surgery in which a long incision started from one side of her jaw, extended continuously behind her hairline, and around to the other side of her jaw. Everything had been laid open with the doctor's sharp scalpel.

Unfortunately, this second surgery was as unsuccessful as the first. The young woman told me the second surgery cost six thou-sand dollars. Both of these surgeries had been performed after my phone conversation with the surgeon. Only recently had she been told there was a physical therapist available who might be able to help her with nonsurgical treatment.

I will admit that I was saddened, disappointed, and more than a bit angry to think that this woman had been subjected to painful and expensive surgeries and had been allowed to continue to suffer all that pain and physical dysfunction for such a long time when the surgeon had known three years earlier that nonintrusive and con-siderably less expensive treatment was available. It was an example of what I call surgical mutilation—that is to say, inexcusable surgi-cal mutilation!

When I examined her, I found that the tissues of her scalp, face, jaw, neck, and upper back were severely tight, contracted, and exquisitely tender to the lightest touch. The surgical scar was eas-ily palpated. Touching it caused additional discomfort. She was in continuous pain, and the slightest movement of her jaw caused the pain to intensify greatly. She told me she was at that moment expe-riencing her constant headache. She spoke slowly, as if she were in severe pain.

I started the two-week course of microcurrent treatment. Unfortunately, it did not produce the results I had hoped for. So at the end of the two-week trial, I phoned the referring dentist and told him that the microcurrent hadn't worked and I was ready to start treatment using my regular techniques.

To my surprise, he told me to stop treatment. He said he had other things in mind. I reminded him that the original plan was a two-week trial of microcurrent and that I was confident I could help this young woman. But he said no, stop treatment.

I was disappointed. My knowledge of the treatments in vogue regarding TMJ led me to believe that this young woman would not be helped and she would continue to suffer severe pain and dysfunction. Nevertheless, I had no choice but to stop treatment.

However, I was haunted by the thought that this young woman was continuing to suffer. Also, once I start treating someone, I become dedicated to achieve success. I felt frustrated and guilty in this case.

After two years had passed, I decided to call the father of this young woman, now twenty, to see how she was doing. Her father told me she was the same. Same headache, same jaw pain, same physical dysfunction. I asked what the dentist had tried after he took me off the case. I learned that the young woman had been sent to a "pain management center" for one visit. She had been given some "pain medication" that hadn't helped her.

I told her father that I had been troubled because I hadn't been allowed to continue to treat his daughter, and if she was interested, I would like to try again. I told him I would not charge for my services, that my only motivation was to help her. I told him I would need a prescription to treat if she decided to try again. He said he would call her and pass on my message.

She called back a few minutes later and said she did indeed want to try again. She said she could get a doctor's prescription, and we set up an appointment for the next day.

When she came in for her treatment, she told me I only had one week to work on her, as she was about to leave the area. When I examined her, I found she still had severely tight and contracted tissues around both sides of her jaw and on around the back of her neck and up into her scalp. All these tissues were extremely painful to light palpation.

I treated her for three consecutive days in two-hour sessions, without any significant response. There was some softening of the contracted tissue and some minimal improvement in jaw opening but no letup in the headache or pain when she moved her jaw.

However, when she came in for her fourth treatment, she told me that she no longer had a headache. It was completely gone. A few hours after the last treatment, the tight areas I had been working on had finally relaxed. In addition, she was now able to open her jaw enough to eat regular food without pain, although she did not have a completely full jaw opening. I only had the opportunity of treating her one more time before she moved away.

I spoke to her by phone one year later. She said that the headache had never returned, her jaw had remained relaxed, and she was continuing to eat regular food without any pain or discomfort. I told her to call me if she had any return of prior symptoms.

Soft Tissue Manipulation Techniques

Soft tissue dysfunction is the primary cause of TMJ pain. The problem is with tight, contracted, fibrotic tissues outside the joint. The pain radiates and is perceived to be coming from within the joint. As with most symptoms of soft tissue dysfunction, TMJ pain is usually an expression of an extensive problem. Look for tight, contracted, and painful tissues in the scalp, face, neck, and upper back. All these areas have to be examined, treated, and normalized. Review the treatment of these areas as described in "Migraine and Muscle Contraction Headaches," "Sinus Headache," and "Sinus Pain."

We will now concentrate on jaw tissue proper, usually the most important contributor of pain and physical dysfunction. The primary muscle that is responsible for chewing action, the masseter, begins just above the joint. It starts as a narrow band and widens as it descends to its attachment on the jawbone. When the masseter contracts, it brings the jaw up so food can be chewed. It is a strong muscle and, when it spasms, it grips your jaw tightly.

A misguided form of treatment is to attempt to force your jaw open. Medical technicians have devices that are designed to do just that, but do not allow this to be done to you. It will stimulate your masseter to become even more painful and dysfunctional; it is a form of torture rather than treatment, and if doctors suggest surgery, tell them to read this book first.

The proper treatment for any soft tissue dysfunction is to soften and normalize the tissue. Soften and normalize the masseter, and it will release its grip on your jaw and your pain will go away.

Start by placing the knuckles of your fingers against your cheek, using your thumb as the probe and treating instrument. Brace the elbow of your treating hand against the wrist of your other hand, which, in turn, is resting against your abdomen. This will give you leverage and prevent fatigue. Begin without lotion. The dysfunction of the masseter is usually so severe that you won't need the lotion to reveal the fibrotic formations, and the friction will allow you to use the skin to assist your probing. You will see what I mean once you try it.

Try circles with the tip of your thumb and then with the pad of your thumb. Alternate this from time to time. Go slowly, as the tissues here need a lot of care. I feel confident that you will immediately find thick, contracted, and fibrotic tissue that contains large amounts of pain. Now apply lotion and continue your explorations.

Move your examining hand so the thumb is placed in a stationary position under your jaw. This allows your forefinger to be used in a free-floating manner to find the outline of the masseter. The muscle is triangular-shaped and attaches to about half of the jawbone. Use your forefinger in side-

Dysfunctioning areas that cause TMJ pain

to-side movements until you get a good idea of the masseter's boundaries, then focus your attention specifically on the muscle. Treat it thoroughly. It will probably be painful to begin with, and will likely become even more tender once you start treating it, especially where it attaches up near the joint. Use single-, double-, and multiple-finger circles, back-and-forths, thumb and finger drags, ripples, and nudges.

Pay close attention to where the muscle attaches above the joint. Use firm double-finger probes, circles, and back-and-forths. Let your fingers follow wherever pain and tightness leads them, which is probably well up into your scalp.

Clench and release your teeth. This action will reveal all the areas of your scalp that are associated with your temporomandibular joint. You will be surprised how extensive this is. These tissues have to be examined, treated, and normalized. Use multiple-finger back-and-forths, circles, and nudges, and treat these areas thoroughly.

Now carefully examine and treat the masseter where it attaches to your jawbone. Double-finger back-and-forths along the length of your jaw will undoubtedly reveal well-defined fibrotic development in the form of hard wirelike configurations running across the length of your jawbone. Follow them under the jawline. Treat the tissues there by pincering with your thumb on the underside of your jawbone and the knuckle of your bent first finger on the other side. The first finger will remain stationary, and your thumb pad will perform circles and back-and-forths. These wirelike formations will require several treatments to become fully normalized.

Turn your attention to the skin overlying your masseter. Use thumb sweeps and skin graspings. Look for thickened, adherent, and painful skin, particularly at the angle of your jaw. Use your thumb for skin rippling and nudgings there.

Response to treatment can vary. Two or three treatments may bring dramatic reduction in symptoms; however, several treatments are usually required to normalize the dysfunctioning tissues that are primarily responsible for the pain and difficulty in proper jaw movement. At times, response can be frustratingly slow, and several weeks or months (at reduced frequency of treatment) are needed to bring the desired results.

Trigger Finger

An individual may find that one of her fingers has developed a tendency to become locked into a bent position when she attempts to grasp an object. Doctors call this problem a "trigger finger." It is another example of the medical profession focusing on one small part of a patient's body to the exclusion of all the others. Doctors do not realize that all areas of their patient's body are marvelously interconnected.

The problem of trigger finger occurs when tissues of the palm become thick and fibrotic and press down tightly on finger flexors. When this happens, finger movement becomes erratic. However, these fibrotic areas are merely a small part of extensive tissue dysfunction. Doctors are unable to see the total picture. All they can see are the fibrotic nodules; the rest of the body is unimportant and out of focus.

The problem of trigger finger occurs when tissues of the palm become thick and fibrotic and press down tightly on finger flexors. When this happens, finger movement becomes erratic. However, these fibrotic areas are merely a small part of extensive tissue dysfunction.

Case History

A professional artist living one hundred miles from Charlottesville heard about my work and called me. She told me she had a painful problem with her right hand, and that it was interfering with her work as an artist. She said her problem had been diagnosed as trigger finger and that it made it difficult for her to hold a brush and paint. She had been sent to a surgeon, a hand specialist, who first injected the area with cortisone, and when that was unsuccessful, had operated on it. Not only was the surgery unsuccessful but it also made the area more painful, and it was more difficult now to hold and manipulate a brush. She asked if I could help her. I told her that I would need a doctor's prescription to check and treat her. She told me that would be no problem, and we made an appointment for later that week.

She arrived at the appointed time, bearing her prescription. The surgeon who had performed the unsuccessful surgery on her hand had refused to write a prescription allowing me to treat, but another doctor had signed one. When I examined her hand, I found that her fingers were swollen and were purplish in color. They moved slowly and stiffly. The skin of her palm was drawn tight. Her skin creases were deep and tender to palpation.

I noted that the surgical scar in her palm was thick, adherent to adjacent tissue, and was painful to mild palpation. I could feel the thickened tissue adherent to her finger flexors that was causing the trigger finger effect. I also found that the tissues extending from her hand up through her arm to her shoulder, neck, and back, were tight, contracted, fibrotic, and extremely painful to palpation.

She responded well to treatment, and in ten sessions the tissues in her hand and fingers, and throughout her upper extremity, were soft, supple, and pain-free. She no longer had symptoms of trigger finger and could paint without any discomfort or disability. She was discharged, healthy and happy.

Soft Tissue Manipulation Techniques

For treatment techniques, refer to "Carpal Tunnel Syndrome."

Weight Loss

The focus of my professional life has been to treat body and headache pain and associated physical dysfunction. The following case history started out with those goals but led to something else that I would like to share with you.

Case History

A woman in her early forties came for treatment because of severe pain throughout her body. She also complained of fatigue and a feeling that her body was getting "tighter." She said she felt her skin was so tight that she was having difficulty moving. She stated that she had to pull herself slowly up stairways by using the stair rails. In addition to all this, she said she was deeply depressed.

When I examined her, I found appreciable thick, contracted, fibrotic tissue throughout her body. She responded well to treatment, and in two weeks her pain was significantly reduced, as was her feeling of fatigue and tightness. However, her depression remained. When we discussed this, she stated that she was depressed because of her "weight problem." She related that when she was married, twenty years earlier, she had a trim figure; her husband could put his hands around her waist, but over the years she had gradually gained too much weight.

She said that for the past two years he had not demonstrated romantic interest in her because she had become "so fat." Formerly, men would glance at her figure; now they paid no attention. She had lost her self-image of being an attractive female. Indeed, her body was rotund and pear-shaped.

Frequently, at this stage of treatment, with pain and other symptoms significantly reduced, I would be thinking about discharge in the near future. However, as I could still feel thick body tissues, I thought there might be a possibility that if they could be reduced, then perhaps her body contours might also be reduced. I discussed this with her. I told her that I could not offer a guarantee that we would be successful, but that it might be worth a try. She said to go ahead.

I continued to work intensively wherever I felt those thick, fibrotic tissues. And here is when an interesting treatment pattern developed. I would work for forty minutes, then she would excuse herself to go to the lavatory. She returned to state that she had voided a large amount of urine. Another forty minutes, followed by another large voiding. This treatment dynamic continued in two-hour sessions, three times a week, for the next eight weeks. At the end of this time, to my astonishment and her delight, she once again had a trim figure. She was then discharged from treatment, pain-free, slim, and happy. I chanced to meet her two years later. She still looked trim and stated that she felt very feminine.

Soft Tissue Manipulation Techniques

The above case history is the only one in which I directed my treatment techniques primarily toward weight or shape reduction. I have treated many other patients who benefited cosmetically from tissue manipulation, but those benefits were derived concurrently with the efforts to treat the pain they were experiencing. Once the pain problem was solved, they were discharged from treatment. For example, while treating the face and neck for areas of tissue dysfunction, patients told me that their friends had asked if they had lost weight recently. One woman, whose neck had lost thick folds, reported that friends thought she had received cosmetic surgery.

Here is my suggestion for self-treatment. Explore the area of your body that you desire to lose weight or reduce contour. Refer to the treatment section that corresponds to that area for treatment techniques. If you find areas of hidden pain and thick, fibrotic tissue, continue treating. If you do not find signs of tissue dysfunction, I would be inclined to think that the area instead contains stored fat, and that diet considerations and increased activity would be the better approach.

Whiplash and Other Accident Trauma

Soft tissues of the body immediately react to the trauma of a motor vehicle accident by going into spasm. Once spasm starts, it never releases, and becomes self-perpetuating. Spasmed tissue is the initiator of progressive pain and physical dysfunction, because unless properly treated, it gradually becomes contracted and then fibrotic.

In addition, as time passes, the local area that was originally injured triggers other areas of the body to become affected, so what was once a limited local problem becomes extensive and global. Unless properly treated, the pain and physical dysfunction that follow a motor vehicle accident becomes what doctors call chronic.

If spasmed tissue is properly treated and released early on, the later stage of contraction and fibrosis can be avoided. The earlier effective treatment is initiated, the easier the problem is to treat, and the greater the assurance for a successful outcome.

However, even the late stage of development, the so-called chronic stage, responds to proper treatment. That is to say, even when body tissues have been allowed to become severely contracted and fibrotic, expectation of significant reversal of tissue dysfunction and its secondary symptom of pain is still high, although these cases are more challenging to treat.

I have frequently heard the comment, "Once you've been in a car accident, you're never the same again." Unfortunately, this is usually true, but if proper treatment is given, it doesn't have to be.

I will describe two cases, one in which timely treatment was given, and the other in which it wasn't, that make this point clear.

Case History 1

A young woman was referred for treatment four days after her car was rear-ended. She presented with severe pain and tightness throughout her neck, back, chest, and both arms. She experienced severe and constant headaches. She was anxious and tearful and found it difficult to concentrate. Going into work was agonizing because of the severe pain, which worsened as the day went on.

When I examined her, I found that the tissues of her scalp, neck, back, upper chest, and both arms were severely spasmed and painful to even very mild palpation. She said she was experiencing a very severe headache. She talked and moved slowly, as if she were in severe pain.

I treated her gently for two hours. I could feel the spasm reducing as I worked. At the end of the two-hour treatment, her headache was almost gone, her body pain was "a lot less," and she felt "much, much, better."

I continued to treat her, at decreasing frequency, for five weeks. At the end of this time, she was symptom-free, she had no body or headache pain, and her tissues were soft and supple. She was discharged, happy and delighted.

Case History 2

A woman was referred to me two years after she had been injured in a motor vehicle accident. She also had been involved in a rear-end collision. She told me she had been treated with pain and anti-inflammatory medication. Her doctor had also prescribed a course of physical therapy consisting of hot packs, five minutes of massage, four or five minutes of ultrasound, and exercises and stretches. Her condition worsened as these treatments continued. By the end of each physical therapy session, her pain became "almost unbearable."

After four months of these treatments, her pain had developed into a constant agony. She couldn't bear another physical therapy session, and so she stopped going. She was criticized by her doctor and physical therapist for being "noncompliant," and this observation was duly noted in her medical record.

Since that time, she required as much pain medication as her doctor would allow, just to "barely survive." She was depressed, in constant pain, had frequent, severe headaches, and was at risk of losing her job because of frequent work absences. She was very concerned because her pain, unbearable as it was, was gradually getting worse and her body was getting ever tighter.

When I examined her, I found that the tissues of her scalp, neck, back, chest, and both arms were tight, thick, contracted, and fibrotic. The skin overlying these areas was thickened, adherent to underlying tissues, and was exquisitely tender to even the lightest touch.

Immediately following a very mild first treatment, her body reacted with a flare-up of excruciating pain throughout the treated area. It was one hour before things calmed down enough for her to leave my office. I apologized for the increased pain the treatment had caused, but she told me she was encouraged because her body felt a little "looser," and she could move a "little easier."

Following the first few treatments, she experienced increased pain, but at the same time, she noticed that her tissues felt looser and lighter. As treatments continued, she no longer experienced increased pain; instead, her body and headache pain lessened during and after each treatment.

I treated her in two-hour sessions, three times a week for the next three months. Gradually, her tissues became less thick, fibrotic, and painful. She was no longer missing work, and her quality of life had improved dramatically. I wanted to continue treating her, to normalize the significant areas of tissue dysfunction that remained, but she had to move away from the area.

I called her a year after treatments stopped. She told me she was doing "so-so." She could feel her body gradually retightening and had tried to find somebody in her area that treated the same way I did, but had been unsuccessful.

It is unfortunate this woman's body had been allowed to become severely contracted and fibrotic. If proper and effective treatment had been started early, it is likely that her pain and suffering could have been avoided.

Soft Tissue Manipulation Techniques

The primary areas to be treated for whiplash are the head, neck, upper back, and chest. Review "Migraine and Muscle Contraction Headaches" for instructions. If other areas of your body have been injured in a car accident, refer to the corresponding treatment sections.

Afterword:

The Healthcare of the Future

As the cases and instructions in this book show, soft tissue dysfunction is the primary cause of body and headache pain, from migraines to painful bunions. Physical and emotional insults stimulate the body to form contracted tissues that squeeze pain receptors and derange joint structures. The process starts in early childhood and progresses throughout the life of the individual.

The cause of body and headache pain can be treated and normalized so pain and its accompanying physical disorder will go away and stay away. The sooner treatment is initiated, the more likely a complete reversal will occur. Sadly, the system of care presently in place does not provide treatment for any stage of this process.

A new healthcare system is needed, one that recognizes and treats tissue dysfunction, instead of dispensing costly drugs and drastic surgeries directed toward its secondary symptoms.

In the future, pain sufferers will not have to treat themselves. I envision a system that provides periodic "tissue checks." Practitioners will carefully examine the body from head to toe. They will look for, identify, and treat *early* stages of spasm, before the health of the individual is compromised, *before* pain occurs.

This will make for a healthier and happier population. There will be enormous savings because costly drugs, surgeries, and the currently unproductive and repetitive provider visits will be eliminated. Individuals will be treated by practitioners who charge reasonable fees for good, honest work, instead of paying exorbitant fees to so-called experts and high-priced surgeons.

For example, an article titled "What Is Carpal Tunnel Syndrome?" that appeared in the July 14, 1999, issue of *The Journal of the American Medical Association* (vol. 282, no. 2) states, "More than 200,000 carpal tunnel release surgical procedures are performed each year in the United States, which makes it the most common surgical procedure performed on the hand."

> In the future, pain sufferers will not have to treat themselves. I envision a system that provides periodic "tissue checks." Practitioners will carefully examine the body from head to toe. They will look for, identify, and treat early stages of spasm, before the health of the individual is compromised, before pain occurs.

The article points out that these procedures, estimated to cost more than one billion dollars per year, are performed without a clear diagnostic basis.

This means that in the next five years doctors will cut into one million carpal tunnels, at a cost to society of five billion dollars, yet all without diagnostic justification!

The practitioners of the healthcare of the future will look back at this period as the dark ages of body and headache pain treatment. By keeping tissues healthy, symptoms of carpal tunnel syndrome that now occur in epidemic proportions will be a thing of the past. Billions of dollars will be saved by changing our treatment approach for this one condition alone.

Think of the many thousands of surgeries performed every year on necks, backs, hips, and knees that are directed toward the *secondary* symptom of pain without any regard to the problem that caused the pain and continues to undermine the health of the pain sufferer after the inappropriate surgery has been performed. Here, we will get into astronomical amounts of savings because inevitably the global aspects of tight, contracted body tissues profoundly degrades the health of the pain sufferer, and the resulting costs to society from conventional but ineffective treatments are incalculable.

It is my contention that the majority of people who end up in nursing homes, wracked with pain and unable to take care of themselves, are there because their bodies became progressively dysfunctional over a period of years, because conventional doctors were unable to provide effective remedies. This is the end result of the present misguided and inappropriate healthcare system.

The practitioners of the future will understand the relationship between soft tissue dysfunction and organ systems that results in a lowered level of health. I have caught glimpses of this relationship. For example, I have observed central blood pressures drop significantly, for extended periods, by softening contracted tissues of the low back and gluteal region. This demonstrates a relationship between soft tissue dysfunction and the cardiovascular system. And if there is a relationship with the cardiovascular system, why not, then, with other systems of the body?

I believe the importance of treating soft tissue dysfunction early in life, before extensive damage takes place, before organ systems are affected, will be appreciated and acted upon, and the present methods of mistreating soft tissue dysfunction with drugs and mutilating surgery will be completely discredited. You will go to a practitioner who understands how your body works, and who knows the soft tissue manipulation techniques that will keep you healthy and free of pain. I hope this book points the way to that healthcare of the future.

For Further Information . . .

Do you have anecdotes of how you were treated for your body or headache pain that you would like to share? If so, I would like to hear from you. Visit my website and send feedback at *www.TissueSculpting.com* or write to me in care of Hampton Roads Publishing Company.

Index

About the Author

Bernard Schatz, P.T., has been in physical therapy practice since 1957. Schatz supervised the Cardiovascular Research Laboratory at Cedars of Lebanon Hospital in Los Angeles, and has worked as staff physical therapist and supervisor in acute hospitals, extended care facilities, and nursing homes. In addition to maintaining a successful private practice, he owned a large rehabilitation company and served as the administrator of a home health agency. Schatz is also a talented artist, entertainer, satirist, and folk singer who has appeared on the Steve Allen and Regis Philbin shows. He lives in Charlottesville, Virginia.

Hampton Roads Publishing Company

. . . for the evolving human spirit

Hampton Roads Publishing Company
publishes books on a variety of subjects,
including metaphysics, health, integrative medicine,
visionary fiction, and other related topics.

For a copy of our latest catalog, call toll-free
(800) 766-8009, or send your name and address to:

Hampton Roads Publishing Company, Inc.
1125 Stoney Ridge Road
Charlottesville, VA 22902

hrpc@hrpub.com
www.hrpub.com